Seeds of Change

A Path to Health and Healing

Laura Dankof, MSN, ARNP, FNP-C
www.pathtohealthandhealing.com

Edited by Penny Fletcher
www.pennyfletcher.com

Cover designed by Rachel Dankof

Seeds 4 Change: A Path to Health and Healing

Copyright © 2013 by Laura Dankof, MSN, ARNP, FNP-C

All rights reserved. No part of this publication may be reproduced or transmitted in any form, or by any means, without written consent from the author, except in the case of brief quotations embodied in reviews.

ISBN-13: 978-1481929660

ISBN-10: 1481929666

www.pathtohealthandhealing.com

Disclaimer

Seeds 4 Change is for educational and informational purposes only and is not a substitute for seeking medical attention when necessary. This book is designed to be an adjunct to your health and healing. The information in this book is not a replacement for seeking appropriate health care advice from a licensed health professional. Please consult your health care provider as needed. The author has made every effort to make sure the content in this book is as accurate and complete as possible. No warranty may be extended or created on these materials. Neither the author nor the publisher shall be liable for any damages including and not limited to incidental, consequential, or any other damages from reading this material.

TABLE OF CONTENTS

Introduction	5
Chapter 1: Planting the seed	10
Chapter 2: Sleep	20
Chapter 3: Environment	36
Chapter 4: Exercise	52
Chapter 5: Diet	62
Chapter 6: Supplements	87
Chapter 7: 4 undiscovered pathways to health: Stress, Gastrointestinal Health, Detoxification, and Hormones	117
Chapter 8: Change	179
Chapter 9: Tree of Life	190
Chapter 10: Transformation	216
Recommended Readings	220
References	223
Index	244

Introduction

What does health and healing mean to me? I think this is a question we have all asked ourselves at one time or another. Do you ever feel that your path to obtaining a healthier life is derailed by one obstacle after another? I think we have all felt this way. One of the biggest obstacles often voiced is that there just isn't enough time. Our lives have become so busy and we are constantly being bombarded by information overload, tasks to complete, family, jobs, and bills to pay. How are we to find time to take care of ourselves?

I have worked in health care for many years, first as a nurse and then a nurse practitioner. I remember in my first Nursing 101 class that nursing means "to care" and caring means attending to the whole person's physical, mental, emotional, spiritual, and environmental needs.

This definition of nursing has always been a guiding force for me throughout my career. One of my greatest frustrations over time is that the art of nursing and the art of caring are being lost. As we all have become painfully aware, health care costs are on a runaway train. Governmental and private insurance govern many of our health care decisions. How do we put the brakes on out of control health care costs and gain control of our own health? I firmly believe the way to do this is by taking charge of our own health. This does not mean firing your health care provider or dropping your insurance coverage. It does mean that you and your health care provider need to understand that the path to health and healing is about addressing the whole person. It is not solely about a symptom, labeling a diagnosis, or finding a pill to cover both of these in accordance with what your insurance will pay for. It is about you. How are you going to take back control of your health?

To simply say if I eat healthier and exercise I will be healthy is being naïve. People who do just that still get sick, develop disease, and are running on empty. Why is this? Because staying healthy involves much more than a healthy diet and exercise. It is much more than taking a pill for a symptom.

As a nurse practitioner I often feel frustrated about how far off track our health care system has become. Don't get me wrong, modern medicine has saved many lives using modern technology and the latest treatments and life-saving medications. However, when it comes to prevention and engaging you, the patient, as an active partner we have fallen short. I would often hear from my patients the concerns about the cost of health care, their concerns about the side effects of medications, and their feeling that they are being rushed through their appointments and not being listened to. They are so appreciative when they feel they are being listened to and actually heard. Often a patient is asking "why have I become ill and how do I get better," not solely what medication is going to fix the problems I am having.

This is where health care has gotten off track, by adopting a mentality of focusing on a symptom and finding a corresponding pill to treat the symptom, instead of asking why. Why does the patient have the symptom? I firmly believe if we as health care providers stop long enough to listen to you, the patient, that you will tell us exactly what is wrong and give us clues to the root cause of your illness or disease.

It is my hope that this book will increase your awareness of how powerful you can be in affecting your own health and the quality of your life. The root of illness and disease do not come by chance or genetics alone, but are affected by multiple factors and certainly are not resolved by simply taking a pill. "Seeds 4 Change" is designed to address many of the factors that are at the root of poor health and disease and to help you find your own path to health and healing.

Taking steps to improve one's health can seem like an overwhelming task, particularly when all our lives are so busy. By taking things one step at a time, no matter how long it takes you can get there. This book is designed to help you address those factors that can change your health and well-being. Just planting one seed and nurturing the soil, in this case your body will help establish a healthy root system. This will allow that seed to have the best chance to grow into a strong, beautiful tree. That tree is you and it is your life. The tree of life symbolizes knowledge. Knowledge is power and having the knowledge you will gain here can significantly impact your quality of life moving forward.

Make an appointment now with yourself to care for your physical, mental, emotional, spiritual, and environmental needs. By doing so you can plant the seed to change and transform your life.

I wish you the very best along this journey and hope that in some small way this book helps you along that path.

    Sincerely,

    Laura Dankof, MSN, ARNP

Acknowledgements

I want to thank my family who has supported me throughout my life both personally and professionally. I would also like to thank all the mentors, teachers, colleagues, and patients that have fostered my professional growth and development. All of you have helped shape who I am today.

CHAPTER ONE

Planting the Seed

I grew up on a small farm in the Midwest. I remember my dad having the soil tested before planting the crops and also rotating the crops that were planted each year. One year he planted corn in the field and the next year beans. It was important that the soil contained the right nutrients and minerals for the plants to grow. Once the seeds were planted and for the crops to be successful they required constant attention to make sure they would remain viable.

They needed water, sun, nutrients, and protection from disease, weeds, and bugs. Otherwise the plant could wither and die. If a problem developed with the plant my dad would look to diagnose the problem. Had something changed in the soil? Had a parasite infected the plant? Was there damage to the root system? He would try to get to the root of the problem so that he could diagnose the underlying cause and fix it.

A farmer's crop is his bread and butter. If my dad would have thought maybe the crop just needs more water, less sun, or more fertilizer. If he had done any of these things without first looking for the underlying cause, he may well have killed the crop and his income for the year. If he did not adjust to changes in the environment that were affecting the plants and had believed the only way to help them grow was by simply watering them, he would not have lasted long as a farmer.

Our health and well-being is a lot like farming. If we don't tend to the soil, (our bodies) we are more likely to develop disease and wither and die at a more accelerated rate, not unlike a field of corn or beans. If we nurture and care for ourselves we can grow to full maturity and a long and healthy life.

If an illness develops, throwing fertilizer on it such as drugs, alcohol, poor eating habits to name a few, we are only masking the problem and may accelerate whatever is ailing us. So I challenge you to ask yourself, what is at the root of the problem? What has affected the quality of your soil, in this case your body, mind and spirit? How do I get things back into balance with the right nutrients and minerals and plant the seed for change? How do I turn things around so that I am not withering on the vine? Like the farmer you must take time to attend to your crop or your body's needs along with your mental and emotional needs. If we don't, the chances of developing illness and disease become more likely.

What you are about to learn is that in order to change the path you are on you must first accept that there is something that needs to be changed. This can be scary, but is liberating as well. No one gets through life without making adjustments to their environment. We all experience change on a daily basis at some level. Sticking your head in the sand or remaining in denial about what is going on with your lifestyle choices and not being able to adapt to the world around you will only leave you stuck.

All of us are who we are because of the experiences we have had in life and the choices we make. We can remain locked in fear or we can break free and start living instead of simply existing. Like many of you reading this book I was locked in fear for much of my life. I was afraid to take risks, afraid of what others would think of me. I was afraid of failing or having others see me fail. Then, like many who have chosen to take control of their life and not be a victim of life, I had a life-altering experience that gave me the strength and courage to step out of the fears that were holding me in place. I learned to embrace what I was called to do in this life. I knew my purpose was to work as a teacher and healer. I did not want to face this calling, out of fear. So what was the life-altering experience that made me face my fears head on? It was the birth and death of my son.

Back in 1989 my husband and I were expecting our second child. When I was approximately thirty-four weeks pregnant I went into preterm labor and found out I was carrying a boy. However this boy, our son, had a non-survivable birth defect. His kidneys never formed. We were devastated. The preterm labor was stopped and genetic tests followed. We felt like we were in the middle of a nightmare. Two weeks later I went into labor again. I did not want labor to come, because I knew that the life I was carrying and feeling move inside me would end with his birth. Our beautiful boy was born on June 6, 1989. He looked just like his father. We held him and cried for hours.

Letting him go was the hardest thing I have ever done. I decided at that moment I could either be a victim lost in my own grief or I would learn something from the experience and be a survivor. I decided to fight and give our son meaning. It was at that pivotal moment, in the height of my grief, that I felt I had nothing to lose. I was going to quit worrying about what people thought of me. I faced my fears and went to nursing school. I was going to fulfill the life purpose I was called here to do, to be a teacher and healer.

My son was going to be my anchor of courage. Though his life was very brief, what he taught me will last a lifetime. It changed who I am and how I perceive the world around me. Do I still have fears, sure, but I am living instead of existing. My hope for you is to live in gratitude for what you have, not what you don't have. Resistance to change focuses on the negative. Having gratitude and finding the things in life to be thankful for gives you strength, and courage to transform and grow, like the Tree of Life. I am grateful to have a wonderful husband and two beautiful daughters. I am grateful to have a roof over my head. I am grateful to have oxygen to breathe. I could go on and on.

I only want the best for you. Your health and well-being are important and you are important. We all have a purpose for being here and we all have something to teach one another. We all have room to grow. No one is perfect and no one gets through life without being transformed by our experiences.

The purpose of this book is to help give you some foundational tools to start your own transformation. Be grateful for the good and bad in life and now use those experiences to direct you on a positive path to health and healing on a physical, mental, emotional, and spiritual level. When conceiving the concept for this book, I wanted it to be easy and straight forward. I want you to be able to take away little tidbits that you can apply to your everyday life right now. So instead of talking with you about how we go about making a change as important as our health, I want you to first become aware. Aware as to why sleep, your environment, exercise, diet, supplements, gastrointestinal health, efficient detoxification, and hormonal balance are such a big deal.

These are the roots of your tree of life, meaning your body and soul. By becoming aware you gain a better understanding about why making a healthy lifestyle change is important. It is my hope for all of you that you will then transform your life to one of great joy and abundance.

The cover of the book was designed to reflect how, if we plant that seed of awareness, we can grow into something much grander. The tree that grows from one tiny seed, when loved and nurtured will transform itself into a majestic symbol of strength. The color green that is on the cover symbolizes the heart chakra or healing in the body. It is hoped you will gain insight into the energetic aspects of your spiritual essence and how important that is to living a life of love and gratitude. This will help in healing your emotional wounds that you have been inflicted with in life. Move out of your fear and into who you are meant to be.

Emotional blocks open the path for dis-ease to develop and poor lifestyle habits to continue. I know you are hungry to find answers. We are all energetic beings with thoughts, feeling and emotions. Uncovering our emotional blocks will take more than what conventional medicine can offer you.

The Internet has opened up a world of possibilities and challenges in the area of self- empowerment and health. It is hard to decipher what information is credible. Having access to natural medicine, energy healers, herbalists and other techniques is very important. In an ideal world you would have access to the alternative healing modalities and conventional medicine equally. They all have something to offer to help guide you on your path to health. Would it not be great if they all worked together, collaborating to help you achieve your best?

Unfortunately this is not what happens. To complicate things further you have the influence of governmental over-regulation, pharmaceutical company research-driven bias, and old ways of thinking getting in the way of your health. All of us that work in health care are to have your greatest good at heart and to do no harm. Sadly personal bias and a lack of appreciation for the knowledge, talent and skill each of these modalities offer often is not fully realized or appreciated. It is time for this way of thinking to stop as it could cost you your life.

That is why you must become the master of your own health. But there is hope. All is not lost, as the tide is beginning to change as more and more people are becoming aware and waking up to this fact. It is my hope that someday you will have conventional doctors, naturopathic doctors, chiropractors, acupuncturists, energy healers, herbalists, nutritionists and others all working together without personal bias. It is also my hope that by doing so the emphasis on disease shifts to an emphasis on wellness and looking for the root cause of physical, mental, emotional and spiritual imbalances.

Imagine how runaway health care costs could go down if all people, no matter their financial resources, had access to a variety of healing modalities that could be accessed based on individualized needs? Would that not be fantastic? Right now the reality is unless you have the money to pay out of your pocket, you will be limited by what the governmental or insurance plan will cover. For example, massage is a wonderful technique to help with back pain and stress relief. However, unless you have the money to pay for a massage, your treatment for back pain will be limited. It may leave you reliant on pain medication, lost days of work, poor eating habits and lack of exercise because of the pain. What do you think costs more, a massage or all those other things?

I will be discussing many different ideas for taking control of your own health. Some of them you may not have the money to pay for, but many others you can easily implement without spending a lot.

There is an emerging area in the medical field that has been quietly gaining momentum in the last several years and I believe is on the cusp of a mass explosion due to consumer demand. It is vitally necessary to breakdown the walls of bias that began back in the early Twentieth Century. Our current health care system can't financially sustain the current disease-driven health care model. Consumer demand will start to tip the scale more towards disease prevention and wellness. Like the farmer trying to understand the root cause of disease in his crops, medicine too will start looking harder at the root cause of disease in humans.

Disease means that the body is out of sorts or not at ease for some reason. The emerging area of health care that is designed to address the root cause of disease and most clearly encourages collaboration between all health care modalities is known as "functional medicine."

According to the Institute of Functional Medicine, functional medicine is a "personalized medicine that deals with primary prevention and underlying causes instead of symptoms for serious chronic disease," (The Institute of Functional Medicine). Functional medicine is looking for the root cause of disease and addresses many of the aspects that will be touched on in the following pages. The practice of functional medicine allows the patient time to tell the practitioner what is wrong with them and the practitioner time to listen. From there the practitioner can start putting the pieces of the puzzle together that led to the patients' dis-ease or illness.

It means considering how sleep deprivation, the environment, lack of exercise, poor diet and nutrition, and stress impact our functional health. This in turn leads to imbalances in hormone and gastrointestinal regulation, detoxification and our mental well-being.

There is a complex interplay that goes on when looking at these various components of health. There is a domino effect taking place. For example, a poor diet can lead to sleep disruption, and decreased energy can lead to lack of exercise. This can go on to lead to gastrointestinal issues such as constipation that create more stress on the body, poor detoxification, and our ability to respond to the environment around us.

The degree to which this all impacts you will be further dependent on how it relates to your genetic predisposition and the length of time and the degree of your exposure.

So in getting back to my nursing roots I hope to help you along the path to addressing your physical, mental, emotional, spiritual, and environmental needs. Only you can transform the state of your health. You have the power within to heal what has become out of balance.

Remember Dorothy in *"The Wizard of Oz?"* Just follow the yellow brick road and you can find your way home. The path to health and healing lies within each one of us. Like the lion that followed Dorothy, we just need to find the courage to start the process. Plant one small seed at a time and you may be surprised at what you can achieve. Your transformation is up to you.

The Tree of Life is a perfect symbol of strength and the diverse elements that ground us in life and how we transform over time. Now move on down your yellow brick road in the pages ahead to see how you have the power to change and strengthen your roots and your health.

CHAPTER TWO
Sleep

In the pursuit to improve health there are several key elements that need to be addressed. We will be touching on many of those elements in this book, the most obvious of these being diet and exercise. I like to use acronyms as a means to learning and remember things. After all, the title of this book, "Seeds 4 Change" was used in this way in naming the chapters of this book. Just look to the content page. I will be sprinkling a few other acronyms in along the way as you follow your own path through the pages you are about to read.

Having said that, let us first address sleep. Sleep is vitally important to our overall health and well-being. Sleep is essential to sustaining life. If one does not get enough sleep, the ability to have the motivation and energy to tackle any other aspect of life will be less obtainable.

Sleep is a time for our bodies to recharge. Sleep provides the time our conscious minds need to rest and to allow our subconscious minds time to process those everyday stresses we face. When a sleep disturbance develops and is not addressed, this can quickly lead to a downward spiral in one's health. Those less than ideal lifestyle habits you were hoping to change suddenly look like a mountain you can't climb. This will then leave you feeling like a failure. So what do you do? You guessed it. You start eating those high calorie, often high sugar or salty foods, depending on your preference. Your fatigue grows, so you don't have the motivation to exercise. The world around you becomes a burden. You gain more weight, your self-esteem plummets and before you know it you are in a physical and emotional warfare with yourself.

Meanwhile the rest of the world is moving on around you and all you want to do is hide. Hopelessness sets in and you don't know how to get the control back into your life. You have become a hormonal and toxic mess. Though this may sound overly dramatic, it illustrates the point, that learning how to get a good night's sleep is one of the first things to address on your path to health and healing.

What is going on in our bodies during sleep? Do you think that you are in the black hole of nothingness? Quite to the contrary, our bodies are very busy. The majority of us will spend about one-third of our life in a sleep state. When looking at the physiology of sleep. There are two types of sleep. They are non-rapid eye movement (NREM) and rapid eye movement (REM). Non-rapid eye movement sleep is where one progresses through to a deeper sleep state.

In the initial phase of sleep there is a period of restful relaxation. This is when what is known as alpha brain waves occur. Sleep then progresses to the deepest sleep state which is known as delta-wave sleep. This is then followed by REM sleep, where dreaming occurs.

While in NREM there is a decrease in brain activity and blood flow. There is also a decrease in heart rate, blood pressure, and body temperature. During REM however there is an increase in blood flow to the motor and sensory areas of the brain, and an increase in heart rate, blood pressure and breathing. During a normal sleep cycle NREM-REM periods will last 70-100 minutes during the first part of the night and up to 90-120 minutes in the later part of the night.

As we age the time spent in REM decreases and NREM increases. This can lead to a poorer quality of sleep and the development of sleep disturbances. This is the result of spending more time in the lighter first half of NREM. Less time is spent in the deeper more restful delta wave half or REM sleep (Colten, Altevogt, 34-37).

It is believed that humans need approximately eight hours of sleep per night. Sadly a large proportion of the population is not getting the necessary eight hours of sleep per night. It would be safe to say that sleep deprivation is likely a national epidemic and health hazard. It is becoming harder and harder to tune out and shut off the distractions of our everyday lives. We are trying to cram in and complete more tasks into our already busy daily lives.

This often includes job, family, recreational activities, cell phones, computers, and television activities to name a few. This results in getting to bed later, waking up earlier, and sleeping less soundly. At some point the body is going to let you know it has had enough. So what are some of the ill effects of long-term sleep deprivation or inadequate sleep? Losing as little as one hour of sleep per night can lead to cognitive decline, decreased immune function, obesity, and increase our risks of heart disease, stroke, and diabetes (Stevens, Benbadis).

Are not obesity, heart disease, stroke, and diabetes some of our top national health concerns? Do you suspect there might be a correlation between sleep and health?

Have you ever known anyone that has been on prednisone for an extended period of time? If you have, you may know that one of the biggest concerns they may have is the amount of weight they are putting on. They may also complain that their blood sugars are high and that they are having trouble sleeping. When you don't get enough sleep, it is like being on prednisone. "Sleep researches from the University of Chicago reported in 2001 that people who slept less than six-and-a-half hours per night secreted fifty percent more insulin and were forty percent less sensitive to the effects of insulin compared to the normal sleeper." More alarming is the fact that by the time we are in our forties we are getting as much as eighty percent less of the deep restful delta wave sleep (Talbott, 96-97, 141-143). The body's adrenal glands respond to this disruption by raising the cortisol levels and disrupting our normal circadian rhythm (Hyman, 169).

Another way to look at this would be like pouring water through a pasta sieve. Clean pure water will filter easily. But what would happen if you added corn syrup? It would start sticking and plugging the holes in the sieve. Less water would be able to get through. When you don't get adequate sleep your cortisol level rises as well as your blood sugar. The pancreas responds by releasing more insulin. Insulin is a hormone that helps to carry the glucose or blood sugar into the cell to be used as energy. As more demands are put on the body it will try to produce more insulin to keep up.

The body is also producing more blood sugar and eventually the system plugs up or can't respond as well. Just like the corn syrup going through a sieve. This is known as insulin resistance. All that excess cortisol and insulin, like the prednisone, has left you fat and tired. Not to mention left you at greater risk for a cascade of health issues.

Insulin resistance equals inflammation. Inflammation along with sleep deprivation opens the door to a host of potential health issues. Cortisol and insulin imbalance can lead to the development of diabetes. Your immune system may become compromised by altering the body's killer T-cell function. This can leave you vulnerable to cancer. Then as hormone function and balance continue to spiral out of control this can lead to mood disturbances and problems with memory and alertness.

Stress hormones may go into overdrive resulting in an irregular heartbeat, high blood pressure and heart disease (Harvard Health Publications). That's not a good way to live.

So what is sabotaging your ability to get a good night sleep? This list could be long and multifaceted. Probably at the top of that list is stress. Stress can make other aspects of life harder to deal with and lessen your sleep quality. Other saboteurs may include physical and mental illness, pain, medications, hormonal fluctuations, snoring, eating late, shift work, and electronics (Belsky). This is by no means a complete list. There are so many things that may be affecting your sleep and ultimately your quality of life.

What is going on in your bedroom? You may have heard it said that there should only be one of two things going on in your bedroom. The first obviously is sleep. The other would be sex. Unfortunately for some, the bedroom becomes a multi-purpose room. It may also serve as an office, a place where you watch television, listen to music, read, and eat. You may have pets that have taken up camp in your bedroom as well. How many electronic devices are clouding your electromagnetic field? With all of this going on, is it any wonder you are having trouble sleeping?

So how do you go about changing your poor sleep habits? First, clear out the clutter, if you are using your bedroom for so many different activities. It is no surprise that you might be having trouble falling asleep or staying asleep. It can be hard to shut off the mind chatter from your day. Having reminders of what you need to do or having a pet interrupt you from a sound sleep are only going to derail your chances at getting a good night's sleep. As mentioned, the bedroom is meant for only two main activities; sleep and sex.

Once you have cleared out the environmental clutter, how do you prepare to go to sleep at night? There may be more to it than visiting the bathroom, brushing your teeth, and saying your prayers like your parents may have taught you growing up. Did your parents give you a set bedtime when you were young? Did you not sleep better when you had a set bedtime? Our bodies are creatures of habit. If you have varying times that you go to bed at night and varying times you wake up, your body will get confused like a baby that mixes up its days and nights.

Inconsistent sleep habits can throw off the normal circadian rhythm. When we go to sleep at night our cortisol levels should be at their lowest and melatonin at its highest. This is important in order for our bodies to relax and fall asleep. This is particularly problematic for shift workers. If you go to bed at 1:00 a.m. one week and 8:00 a.m. another week your body will quickly become confused. So instead of your cortisol being low and melatonin being high, you could have the opposite and it will be extremely difficult to fall asleep and stay asleep.

The golden hours for sleep are 10:00 p.m. to 2:00 a.m. This is when the adrenal glands do their rebuilding and recovery from the day. If you are not asleep at this time, this function can be compromised and can open the door to circadian rhythm imbalance. Getting to bed at 10:00 p.m. may not be a reality or feasible for all people. The key in this case would be to try and have a consistent sleep time and wake time. Even on the weekends.

So what other things can you do to improve your sleep? It is important to have good sleep hygiene practices. By this I don't mean making sure you shower before bed. Though this can certainly be a part of your bedtime preparation.

Sleep hygiene are those things you do to wind down from your day to help you to relax as you prepare to go to sleep. This starts before the golden hour of 10:00 p.m. Try not to eat dinner or consume alcohol after 6 or 7:00 p.m. Limit your caffeine use to before 4:00 p.m. If you are having trouble shutting off your brain, make a "to do list". Journaling may also be helpful. Take a warm bath before bed, meditate, or listen to relaxing music. Try turning the lights down an hour before bed. This will help elevate your melatonin level naturally.

Our bodies naturally produce melatonin, which should be its highest at night. Melatonin helps the body to relax and fall asleep. Try to keep your bedroom cooler. If you are too hot, your body will find it difficult to relax. Remember that during the non-rem cycle of sleep our body temperature is supposed to drop to help us relax and fall into a deeper sleep. If your bed partner snores, try wearing ear plugs or have some white noise such as a fan or nature music like ocean waves going on quietly in the background. Face your alarm clock away from you so you are not waking up and checking the time (Teitelbaum, 49-52).

These simple steps can go a long way to improving your sleep, without the use of over the counter sleep aids or prescription sleep medications.

Let's say you have tried any number of sleep hygiene practices and you are still having trouble falling asleep or staying ould be an underlying medical reason for this and to be evaluated by your health care provider. Any nic illnesses or side effects from medications could be contributing to your poor sleep. You could also be suffering from an undiagnosed sleep disorder. Probably the most common, but also under diagnosed condition is sleep apnea. This is where you can have a few to several episodes where you briefly quit breathing due to obstruction of your airway. Your sleep is consistently unknowingly being interrupted.

This may also be putting stress on your heart and brain as your body is not getting adequate oxygen. People at risk for sleep apnea are those who snore, drink alcohol before bed, are thicker necked, overweight, or have a deviated septum. You may also wake feeling like you have been up all night or awake with a morning headache or dry mouth from sleeping with your mouth open. It is important to have this properly evaluated.

Another common sleep disorder is restless legs syndrome. This is an antsy, uncomfortable feeling in your legs that can occur in the evening or while in bed at night. The discomfort can be relieved by getting up and moving around. Restless legs syndrome may run in families. So you might ask your parents or siblings if any of them are having the same problem. It can also be seen in women that are pregnant, or those that may be suffering from kidney failure, iron deficiency anemia, or peripheral neuropathy (sensation of burning, pins, or needles in your feet often due to other underlying medical conditions). If you suspect you have this condition, talk to your health care provider. If you can identify the underlying cause and treat that, you may gain complete relief from the unpleasantness of restless legs syndrome (Mayo Clinic).

The last sleep disorder I would like to touch on is narcolepsy. This is a rare condition characterized as excessive daytime sleepiness. It can occur at any time and may be triggered by eating a meal, stress, or while driving. There will be an overwhelming urge to fall asleep or take a nap. You may fall asleep in the middle of a conversation. There are different degrees of narcolepsy, some more severe than others. It tends to run in families. In some people narcolepsy has been linked to a decrease production of hypocretin by the brain. There is some belief narcolepsy may be an autoimmune disorder. There are some medications available that may or may not help. It is very hard to treat and your best defense may be making certain lifestyle adjustments such as eating lighter meals during the day, taking a brief nap, and limiting stress if at all possible (National Institutes of Health).

Sometimes in spite of everything you have tried, you are still having trouble getting a good night's sleep. Now what do you do? Psychotherapy is certainly a reasonable option, along with prescription sleep aids. If you can find an integrative or functional practitioner, they can order test to evaluate your hormones, cortisol, and neurotransmitter function. If you correct the underlying imbalance, you may solve your sleep issue. We will talk more about these components in a later chapter.

If you don't have access to a practitioner familiar with functional testing, there are various natural over the counter remedies you can try. I must caution you though, with any remedy, whether herbal, over the counter sleep aid or prescription sleep aid it should be taken only as directed and may interact with other medications or supplements you may be taking. Additionally, if you think taking more than the recommended dose will lead to a greater response you could be putting your own health at risk on any number of levels.

I would also recommend you do your due diligence to research the quality and purity of the product you are purchasing. Speaking to your local pharmacist may be useful as well. They can help you sort out the potential drug to drug or drug to herbal interactions. Having said that lets look at some proven over the counter remedies.

Probably one of the most popular over the counter remedies is melatonin. Melatonin is a hormone our bodies naturally produce and it helps regulate our sleep-wake cycle or circadian rhythm. Endogenous melatonin or the melatonin our body produces naturally, may decrease as we age or with disordered sleep patterns as mentioned earlier. Melatonin has also been found to be useful in preventing and treating symptoms of jet lag. In most studies anywhere from 1-5mg of melatonin was shown to have benefit when taken for up to eight weeks. The mistake most people may make when taking melatonin is taking it right before going to bed. Melatonin works best if you take it one to two hours before bed. This best mirrors the natural rise in melatonin before going to sleep.

Melatonin is not the only natural sleep aid available. For some, they may have no response to melatonin. It really is a matter of trial and error. What may work for one person, may not work well for another. Another option that is increasing in use is 5-Hydroxy-L-Tryptophan or 5-HTP. 5-HTP is an amino acid and precursor to the neurotransmitter serotonin. Often prescribed anti-depressants and anxiolytics are used to slow the uptake of serotonin and thus affect mood. 5-HTP actually encourages the production of serotonin. It can be helpful for those suffering from sleep disturbances that are associated with underlying depression and/or anxiety. It is also frequently recommended by functional practitioners who treat patients with fibromyalgia.

If you are currently taking a prescription anti-depressant, it is important to first talk to your health care provider before taking this product. The recommended dose of 5-HTP is 100-200 mg one to two hours before bed. Taking it with four ounces of grape juice may actually enhance its affect in crossing the blood brain barrier.

Another amino acid that may be used to help you sleep is Gamma-amino butyric acid (GABA). GABA has anxiolytic and sedative properties. GABA may be useful if you are having trouble relaxing enough to fall asleep. If you are having trouble "shutting off your brain", GABA may be worth a try. This should be taken right before bed and doses generally range from 500-1,000mg.

Valerian is an herbal remedy that has been shown to improve overall sleep quality in poor sleepers. It is believed to help one fall asleep faster and provides a deeper more restful sleep. It appears to have the best results when used consistently for an extended period of time versus on only an occasional basis. Valerian is best taken thirty-to-sixty minutes before bed. A clearly defined dosage recommendation has not been determined. Most products contain 300-1,800mg of Valerian. The best available studies have shown that taking 600mg one hour before bed to be sufficient. However, another study showed that taking as little as 180-360mg of valerian in combination with lemon balm improved deep sleep.

A lesser known herbal remedy sometimes used for sleep is Hops, a plant that is a member of the hemp family and may be more familiar to beer drinkers. Now that does not mean that I am suggesting you have a can of beer before bed. In this form, it will likely disrupt your sleep. The Hops plant is believed to have a mild sedative affect and to help with mild anxiety and insomnia. Hops 300-400mg seems to work best when combined with valerian 240-300mg. You can likely find this in a combination herbal sleep remedy.

If you suffer from anxiety that is affecting your sleep, then passionflower may be worth a try. Passionflower has a calming affect similar to acute anxiety medications. However, the scientific evidence on this is not yet completely clear. Passionflower may be found in herbal teas. It can also be found in extract or tincture form. A clear standardized dose has not been established (Teitelbaum; Natural Standards Database).

Essential oils are growing in use for many medicinal purposes. Essential oils are concentrated liquids extracted from aromatic plants and have been used for thousands of years. The earliest reference to essential oils is mentioned in the Bible. Their use in the area of sleep and relaxation is growing - or maybe just being rediscovered. What is nice about essential oils is that you can inhale them through a diffuser, dilute them in carrier oil such as almond oil or olive oil or apply them directly to the skin. Breathing in an essential oil encourages slow deep breathing and natural relaxation. It also leaves a nice fragrance in the room.

One of the more popular remedies used for sleep is lavender. Lavender can be applied to the soles of the feet, placed in a diffuser, or put a drop on your pillow (Young Living Oils).

Up to this point we have focused on ways to help you to get to sleep at night. What is also important to realize is how various lifestyle habits impact sleep as well. Many of those we will be talking about as we continue to plant the "Seeds 4 Change." Your diet is critically important. How you handle stress. Do you suffer from a chronic health condition or mental illness? Are you taking medications that are altering your sleep? Do you exercise? Are you in pain? Do you have a good mattress? It is hoped that some of the suggestions made here you will find helpful.

Make a list of all the things that are going on in your life that you feel are impacting your sleep. Now determine what things on that list you can change and those things that you can't change. This list may be long and a bit intimidating. Once you have your list of things you can change, number them from the most important to the least important to you. Then start tackling them one by one. If you try to tackle them all at once it will likely cause more stress and you are now not sleeping because of the very exercise that is meant to help you tackle the problem in the first place.

For example, let's say you know that drinking a glass of wine before bed, while watching television, and reading a book may be affecting your ability to settle down and fall asleep at night. It might be too much to ask you to stop all of these activities all at once. So start with one of them. Maybe you decide you can stop watching television in the bedroom. Better yet, remove the television. After a week or even a month of this, you move on to the next item on your list you have identified. Next you quit having the glass of wine right before bed. A few weeks later, you stop reading in the bedroom.

You get the idea. Take things one step at a time and before you know it you are sleeping like a baby who has gotten his days and nights finally straightened out.

Take Away Tips

- Try to be in bed by 10:00 p.m. and strive for eight hours of sleep per night.
- Set a consistent bedtime as often as possible.
- Clear out the room clutter and limit electronic devices.
- No caffeine after 4:00 p.m.
- Try not to consume food or alcohol after 6:00-7:00 p.m.
- Relax with music, meditation, and/or a warm bath.
- Keep your bedroom temperature on the cool side.
- Supplements and essential oils can be used when you need a little extra help getting to sleep.
- If you continue to have problems sleeping, get evaluated by your health care provider.

CHAPTER 3

Environment

Do you ever wonder how the environment around you may be affecting your health? It can be overwhelming if you think about the impact our environment can have on our health and well-being. According to the World Health Organization, environmental health is defined as those external factors to a person, whether they are physical, chemical, or biological that can have a profound impact on our health (Environmental Health).

You would think that if you are living in a modern society that your health risk may be less than those living in a less developed country. In some respects this may be true. In other respects your health may be at even greater risk. This can be due to many factors including but not limited to the Standard American Diet or S.A.D. This is certainly an appropriate acronym.

Americans are eating highly processed, sugar and chemical-laden food. Additionally, most food today has been genetically modified. This has most certainly contributed to our current obesity epidemic. As if that is not bad enough our food is grown in fields laced with pesticides and soil that has been stripped of vital nutrients and minerals. The runoff from these fields and sewage are polluting our water supply.

Most Americans are also being exposed to air pollution in one form or another. If you smoke or live with someone who does your air quality is compromised even further. Living in a technological society with cell phones and electrical power poles rising like skyscrapers across the landscape and electronics in our homes are exposing us to a barrage of electromagnetic fields that are hard to escape. If you are using cosmetics, creams, and lotions these are often chemically derived substances whose names you can't pronounce. This is but a small representation of what we are all exposed to on a daily basis. There is no way to escape these exposures completely.

So how do you begin to protect yourself and your family from the health hazards that are all around you? It is important to educate yourself about what the risks are, not only where you live, but the in world as a whole. If humans don't have clean water to drink and clean air to breathe we will cease to exist. Your local city hall can be one place to start educating yourself about the community in which you live. The other is by visiting the Environmental Protection Agency (EPA) website or speaking to someone from the EPA. But do not rely on this alone. Let your intuition guide you through this process.

The mission of the EPA is to protect the American people from health risks that may occur through natural resources, transportation, agriculture, industrialization, economic growth, other humans, energy, and global and international trade (Environmental Protection Agency). The EPA cannot be everywhere at all times. If you have a concern or witness a potential environmental hazard or violation, notify your local authorities or contact the EPA. Be proactive as it often will take the government years to investigate a complaint and even longer to act on it. So if you are concerned about your drinking water, have it tested. If you feel your home is making you sick, move. I know this sounds extreme. But for some these may be their only options in order to maintain their family's health.

Probably one of the best known cases of an individual citizen taking on a big company for violating environmental health and safety standards; was the story of Erin Brockovich. Ms. Brockovich, along with lawyer Ed Masry, took on the lawsuit against Pacific Gas and Electric. According to the lawsuit this company knowingly was polluting the water supply of Hinkley, California by leaking toxic Chromium into the ground water. In the settlement $333 million in damages was owed to the people of Hinkley (Brockovich). This was a well publicized case, but there are no doubt many cases of lesser known heroes like Ms. Brockovich that you never hear of fighting every day to protect the environment we all share. We all need to do our part to protect our precious resources.

Unfortunately the concern of exposure to a toxic water supply is not isolated to Hinkley, California. Many believe that all the world's water supplies have become polluted and are filled with toxins that can contribute to disease. Even water that is melting from our glaciers was found to have pesticides. How does this happen? This is likely the result of acid rain. According to the EPA, "acid rain occurs when gases react in the atmosphere with water, oxygen, and other chemicals to form various acidic compounds. The result is a mild solution of sulfuric acid and nitric acid. When sulfur dioxide and nitrogen oxides are released from power plants and other sources, prevailing winds blow these compounds across state and national borders, sometimes over hundreds of miles" (EPA).

This means that the pesticides a farmer uses in the Midwest can impact the water supply potentially of someone living in Europe. Having grown up in the Midwest on a farm, I am dismayed at the number of farmers who I grew up with that have succumbed to Parkinson's disease. There have been several scientific studies done showing a link between pesticide exposure and Parkinson's disease (Yu, 38-39).

Pesticides are not the only concern. The water you drink and the foods you eat that are harvested likely contain heavy metals such as lead, cadmium, arsenic, and mercury. Heavy metals toxicity has been linked to a number of health issues including heart disease, cancer, and neurological disease to name a few.

How many health care providers are actually considering or testing for these substances? Sadly I would say very few. It is not even on their radar screen to test for these substances. For example there is a case where a gentleman had liver disease. His gastroenterologist told him there was nothing he could do for him and that his disease was progressive. The gentleman had a young family and did not want to accept his fate and came to see the practitioner trained in functional medicine. One of the things he was checked for was heavy metals. To the alarm of the practitioner, he had a toxic level of arsenic in his urine. He worked in construction and was likely inadvertently exposed. His body was not clearing it out, it was theorized to be due to his liver disease.

Many of this gentleman's other labs were grossly abnormal as well. He also had high liver enzymes, cholesterol, estrogen, and low testosterone. He was placed on a year-long intensive program that included aggressive dietary changes, detoxification and supplementation. After working with him for one year, they were able to get all of his labs into normal ranges, including the arsenic level. Originally his gastroenterologist gave him a poor prognosis, telling him he may have only six months to three years to live. He fought hard to live. At the time of this writing, he is still alive four years later and his disease has remained stable.

Just think of how many people could possibly avert disease if more were aware of the affects of heavy metal exposure to their health?

Another toxin that has grown exponentially over the last several years with the fitness craze in the name of good health and clean water is bottled water. The plastic in your bottle water contains bisphenol A (BPA). Bisphenol A from plastics when broken down is a toxin that pollutes our groundwater and the water of the oceans. This is affecting marine life, a very valuable and precious resource. Studies have shown that BPA can affect fertility and hormone balance. There is also research going on looking at a possible association of BPA and breast cancer (Fuchs,

1-3). So in the name of good health we are compromising all life forms.

Replace your plastic water bottle with glass or stainless steel if at all possible. You will not only decrease your exposure to potentially harmful BPA, but the planet as a whole.

One area that probably brings up the most controversy and is supported by the EPA is the deliberate act of adding chlorine and fluoride to our water supply. These substances are placed in our water supply in order to kill bacteria and promote healthy bones and teeth. However, chlorine and fluoride may actually be creating far bigger health hazards. Chlorination of drinking water has been linked to an increase risk of cancer. The cancers that show a correlation with chlorination include: Hodgkin's disease, bladder, colorectal, breast, and esophageal cancer. It has also been associated with male infertility and diseases of the circulatory system.

This is due to a process known as oxidation that occurs when the chlorine interacts with the organic contaminants in the water. Oxidation creates inflammation and where there is inflammation there is greater risks for disease to manifest. Think of it as your system rusting out (Fluoride & Chlorine). When you see pipes and cars that rust, what happens? They start to fall apart. The same thing can happen in the body with excessive oxidation.

Fluoride is another known toxin that is put into our drinking water. Fluoride has been linked with cancer and thyroid disease. There does seem to be an explosion of thyroid disease.

Likely you or someone you know has been affected by this condition, most notably hypothyroidism. Could there be a connection between the upswing in thyroid conditions and fluoride? Many think so.

One of the biggest opponents in a growing movement to ban fluoridation from our drinking water is Dr. Paul Connett, a chemist trained in environmental chemistry. Dr. Connett when interviewed by Dr. Joseph Mercola in the January 29, 2012 online Huffington Post was asked to share his views on this matter.

In that interview, he said, "First of all, water fluoridation is very bad medicine because once you put it in the water, you can't control the dose. You can't control who gets it. There is no oversight. You're allowing a community to do to everyone what a doctor can do to no one, i.e., force a patient to take a particular medication."

Before 1945, when communal water fluoridation in the United States took effect, fluoride was actually listed as a known toxin. Dr. Connett goes on to point out that in regards to tooth decay, fluoride works from the outside of your teeth, so why are we swallowing it? He further notes that there is no difference in the amount of tooth decay between countries that do and countries that do not fluoridate their water supply.

Fluoridation can also cause dental fluorosis which damages the surface of the teeth resulting in discoloration and mottling of the teeth. It has been shown in several studies to lower the I.Q. in children when they were exposed to as little as 1.9 parts per million (ppm) of fluoride. The EPA currently allows up to 4 ppm of fluoride. In 2003, the National Research Council appointed one of the most balanced and objective panels of experts to objectively investigate fluoride and brought this to the attention of the EPA. The EPA has not yet acted on this recommendation.

There is a sad irony in how fluoride is classified. It all depends on how it is being used. Dr. Connett states that fluoride is a substance known as lexafluorosilicic acid or silicon fluoride used to make phosphate fertilizer produces toxic gases of hydrogen fluoride and silicon tetrafluoride. Captured gases when sprayed with water produce silicon fluoride. This toxin Dr. Connett goes on to say could not be dumped into the sea by international law. So how do you get rid of this toxic material? You put in the drinking water.

Here is the sad irony, the EPA states that this substance is a pollutant when found in the air and water, but when your local water utilities put it deliberately into your drinking water it miraculously is no longer a pollutant and is claimed to provide certain health benefits instead of health hazards. The United States is one of only eight countries that allow the fluoridation of water to continue (Mercola). Deliberate fluoridation of the water supply has been banned in many countries due to its potential carcinogenic and toxic effects.

But all is not lost. There are things you can do to protect yourself and your family. Increasing awareness is part of the solution. You can contact your legislatures with your concerns.

Check out resources such as the "Fluoride Action Network." You can place filters on your water tap. This would include your shower heads. You can install a water ionizing or reverse osmosis unit. If you can't afford this, then at the very least consider water purification filter pitcher. These are fairly inexpensive and readily available.

We all know that water is essential to life. The other thing that we must have to survive is oxygen in the air we breathe. What is the quality of your air supply? Are you immune from air pollution if you live in a rural community? If you live in a large metropolitan area you are no doubt familiar with air pollution in the form of smog- that thick haze that hangs over the city.

You may think you are safe once you are locked up nice and tight in your home, however the quality of the air in your home also likely has some form of air pollutants. I don't think there is any argument that since the dawn of the industrial revolution in the Twentieth Century, our air quality has been greatly compromised.

In 1970 the "Clean Air Act" was enacted to ensure the safety of the air we breathe. It is obvious that a lot of work is yet to be done to enforce this act. Poor air quality is a serious health concern. In August 2011 a letter of consensus from several health and medical groups including the American Academy of Pediatrics, American Heart Association, American Lung Association and others was sent to the EPA. In that letter they urged the EPA to "adopt the strongest possible standards to reduce mercury and air toxins from coal and oil-fired power plants.

Most health and medical professionals who treat patients impacted by lung, cardiovascular, and neurological impairments are all keenly aware of the harmful health effects of air pollution. Research has shown that these toxins are especially dangerous because of the harm they cause to the circulatory, respiratory, nervous, endocrine, and other essential life systems within humans. Toxic emissions can even cause developmental disorders and premature death. They went on to urge the EPA to close the two-decade old loophole that has allowed power plants to avoid having to clean up, unlike all other industries. This is a move that is long overdue in the name of public health" (American Lung Association). We can only hope that the EPA takes these concerns seriously and takes action.

Indoor air pollution is also of great concern. Our homes are likely full of toxic chemicals in the form of building materials, cleaning products, and even seeping up from the ground in the form of radon gases that have been linked to lung cancer (University of Iowa). The health risks associated with building materials was brought to our attention when people displaced after hurricane Katrina were given temporary housing in trailer homes.

Residents claimed they were suffering various illnesses, particularly respiratory illnesses, due to the off gassing from formaldehyde. There are ways you can protect yourself and your family from the off gassing of potential hazardous building materials. By using low volatile organic compounds (VOC) paints, carpets, and ecologically-friendly building materials. You want to make sure your home is well ventilated and consider installing high-efficiency particulate air (HEPA) filters.

Instead of buying expensive solvents and chemicals to clean your house, use natural cleaning agents such as water, vinegar, and baking soda to name a few. You can also help your body clear toxic burden by eating a healthy diet rich in antioxidants; particularly those food sources rich in beta carotene, vitamin C, vitamin E, and selenium (Weil, 157-161).

Many of the pollutants we have discussed up to this point may also be referred to as xenobiotics or persistent organic pollutants (POPs). It is believed that since the end of World War II more than 80,000 new POPs have been introduced into our environment. Our bodies do not know what to do with these agents and given the right body stressors and genetic mix they can lead to harmful health effects.

Many studies have shown a correlation between POPs and their impact on our health including threats to our immune system, cancers risks, reproductive and endocrine systems. It is important to try and limit your exposure as much as possible (Bland, 147-150). We know something is affecting us. Girls are developing secondary sex characteristics (breasts, pubic hair, and menstrual cycle) at a younger age. There seems to be a higher incidence of infertility and other hormone-related issues in our younger population.

In the name of beauty, youth and vitality many women and men will slather their bodies in various lotions, cosmetics, and tonics. Do you really know what it is you are putting on your skin? Do you know the potential effect these remedies may have on your health? Many of the beauty products you are spending your good hard cash on may contain sodium laurel sulfate, PEG-30 dipolydrydroxysterate, PEG-120 methyl glucose dioleate, mineral oil, diethanolamine, triethanolamine, methylparaben, propylparaben, diazolidinyl urea, red dye 3 and yellow dye 5.

Unless you are a chemist you likely will have a hard time pronouncing or understanding what any of these ingredients are or their potential health implications. Some of the reported action and effect of these agents are they can strip your skin of their natural oils and actually dry out your skin. Some are derived from petroleum. Others can lead to skin and eye irritation and can even form nitrosamines which can be toxic to the cardiovascular, respiratory and digestive systems.

Most concerning of all, some of these agents has the ability to disrupt hormone balance, better known as estrogen disruptors and potentially increase your risk of cancer. Parabens are the most known for this. So if you see an ingredient with paraben listed, avoid it. There are plenty of safer alternatives available that are chemical free. Do your research and choose wisely. Look for agents that are paraben-free, contain no artificial coloring or fragrance, are hypoallergenic, gluten-free and contain no mineral oil or petroleum based ingredients (Fuchs).

Let's assume you have taken steps to protect your drinking water, are using air filters, and have thrown out all the toxic makeup and cleaning supplies. You may think you are in the clear and have greatly decreased your body's potential toxic burden. Certainly this is a great improvement. However there is another area that is often overlooked and will be much harder to give up.

Are we all not "connected" in some way in this technological age? It would be hard to find someone who does not have a cell phone, television, computer, or any number of electronic devices in their home. So why should you worry about using these devices? I know you are saying there is no way I am going to give up my cell phone or computer. I am not asking you to. Just know your risks and take action to decrease them. There is a great debate within the scientific community as to whether or not electromagnetic fields (EMFs) these devices emit pose any real health risks.

Electromagnetic fields are the exchange between electrical and magnetic charge that are invisible to the naked eye. These can occur naturally in our environment such as what happens during a thunderstorm resulting in thunder and lightning. They can also be man-made such as in an X-ray, cell phone or any number of electrical devices. The radio frequency these devices emit can range from a very low voltage to a very high and immediately deadly voltage on contact (World Health Organization). The amount of EMF we are exposed to today is an astounding one-hundred-million times greater than what our grandparents were exposed to. That is shocking! No pun intended. This exposure may have serious health effects on vulnerable individuals.

Some people are going to be more sensitive to EMF effects than others. It is believed that EMFs have an impact on the pineal gland in our brains and turn on stress hormones in the body. This can result in hormone disruption, in particular melatonin which affects are sleep-wake cycle and our immune system. Low melatonin level has been linked to fibromyalgia, Alzheimer's, Parkinson's, and cancer. Chronic exposure to EMFs can also rob our bodies of essential nutrients vital to reduce oxidative stress and a healthy immune system.

So what can you do to protect yourself and decrease your EMF exposure? You will not be able to eradicate this exposure entirely. You can take steps though to make sure that you have supportive external and internal defenses. The most obvious is to limit your exposure to electronic devices as much as possible. Keep radios, televisions and clocks at least six feet away from your bed, don't use an electric blanket, use LED bulbs instead of compact florescent bulbs, unplug electronic devices you are not using and use a power strip, avoid unnecessary medical tests that use radiation, use an air tube head-set or microphone option when talking on a cell phone and don't carry them next to your skin if possible.

It is also good to consume a diet rich in antioxidants. Examples of foods rich in antioxidants are asparagus, kale, broccoli, cauliflower, cabbage, artichokes, cinnamon, berries, olive oil, and tart cherries. If you want to learn more about the effects of EMFs and what you can do to protect yourself, I would recommend you read *Zapped* by Dr. Ann Louise Gittleman, one of the best known experts of this subject (Fuchs; Gittleman).

After reading about all of the environmental risks you are probably wondering how much any of this has had on your current health. You may also be thinking this is all just too overwhelming to even tackle or that I am healthy and young, why should I worry about it? I don't want you to wake up some day only to hear you have cancer, or a loved one has Parkinson's or Alzheimer's disease.

Be proactive and protect yourself. If you currently are having health concerns there are tests you can have done to evaluate your current body burden. These may include neurotransmitter, heavy metal, hormone, food sensitivity and gastrointestinal analysis through blood, urine, stool and saliva testing. You can also get home test kits to check your water, EMF, radon, mold and other home pollutants. Often these kits can be ordered online or from your local hardware store. Your best defense is knowledge. The more information you have the better you are able to respond to decrease your exposure and potential health risks.

Take Away Tips

- Get your drinking water tested and drink filtered water.
- Place water filters on shower heads to limit chlorine exposure.
- Have your home tested for radon gas.
- Be informed about the quality of air, land, and ground water in your community.
- Quit drinking out of plastic water bottles.
- Use low VOC building materials.
- Install a HEPA filter on your furnace.
- Use natural cleaning products.
- Use organic cosmetics with simple to read ingredients.
- Limit your EMF exposure.

CHAPTER FOUR
Exercise

Arrgghh!!! This may be how you feel when someone mentions exercise. Why are so many people adverse to the thought of exercise? You would think it is a curse word!

Instead of calling it exercise, for some, it is "extra excuses." Are you one of those people that can quickly name off various reasons as to why you don't exercise? I don't have time. I'm too heavy. It hurts to exercise. What does it matter, I am already fat and out of shape. I have tried and I just don't lose any weight. Do any of these sound familiar? Even the granddaddy of exercise, Jack Lalane was quoted as stating he didn't like to exercise. Yet he got up and did it every day until he sadly succumbed to pneumonia at the age of ninety-three.

It certainly was not because he was out of shape. He was an exceptionally fit human specimen. I have to admit I often begrudge exercise myself. I also know the enormous benefits exercise has as well. As a nurse practitioner it is sometimes frustrating to hear all the excuses people use particularly when I know what a profound impact exercise can have on an individual's health and well-being.

There have been numerous studies conducted on the benefits of exercise. Before going into the scientifically proven benefits of exercise let's face the state of denial. At one end of the spectrum you have people that are overweight and out of shape viewing themselves as being indestructible and immune to disease and disability and at the other end of the spectrum are the underweight or normal weight individuals who exercise excessively.

What is the cost of your denial? An alarming sixty-five percent of Americans are overweight and thirty percent of these people perceive they are at a normal weight, while seventy percent of those who are obese perceive themselves as just overweight! If we as Americans continue on this path, it is predicted that by 2020, seventy-five percent of us will be carrying around excess weight.

Think of the personal and financial costs this will have. The economic impact on our out-of-control health care costs is already enormous. In 2011, the annual cost to treat the disease manifestations of overweight and obese individuals was $93 billion! That's right, I said $93 billion! That excess weight is contributing to all of the leading causes of disease and disability including heart disease, diabetes, cancer, stroke, auto-immune disease, arthritis and infection (Faloon, 7-14).

A published report in the December 2010 *New England Journal of Medicine* further illustrates the mortality risks. If you are a woman who is only mildly overweight with a body mass index (BMI) of 25-29 your mortality risk increases by 13%. An obese woman with a BMI of 30-34.9 and your risk goes up to 44% and from 35-39.9 and you are at 88% increased risk. For the growing epidemic of the morbidly obese women your likely risk of dying is a shocking 151%. The findings were similar in men as well (de Gonzalez, Hartge, Cerhand, 2211-2219). Next time you go to your healthcare provider, ask what your BMI is to help motivate you to take action.

Why am I bringing up the issue of obesity here? There is more to being overweight or obese than whether or not you exercise. However one of the many factors that can be keeping you from an optimal life is your weight. Exercise expends energy while inactivity does not and this leads to weight gain. As we age many people will become less physically active further increasing the risk to become overweight or obese. This lack of physical activity can lead to 120-190 extra calories being stored as fat and in one year's time this will equal an extra 13-20 pounds. So in order to keep your metabolic rate up instead of declining as you age, you have got to keep moving (Goepp, 27-35). A consistent program of regular exercise can build muscle and bone thereby increasing our energy expenditure and reducing body fat (Talbott, 145).

So what are the benefits of exercise other than trying to keep your weight in check? Exercise is one of the best ways to help increase your life expectancy. Its impact on our hormonal and nervous systems are enormous. Exercise has been shown to increase growth hormone and testosterone and regulate estrogen and progesterone. It also will help improve insulin sensitivity and decrease your risk of developing diabetes. All these things can affect the aging process. Exercise can help regulate mood by increasing neurotransmitters such as GABA to keep anxiety in check, serotonin and norepinephrine to decrease depression or low mood, and dopamine which has an effect on energy level. It boosts endorphins, which are our body's natural painkiller and mood enhancer.

All of these can affect the ability to respond to stress and enjoy life. You don't just want to extend your life; you want to be of sound mind as well. Exercise has been shown to increase brain-derived neurotrophic factor. This helps to keep neurons functioning and our thought processes working and keeps dementia at bay. Most people have heard of the cardiovascular benefits of exercise as well. It can help to decrease your blood pressure, cholesterol, the stickiness of your blood, inflammation in the blood vessels, and workload on the heart (Hyman, 314-315; Musnick, 483-484).

And there's still more! I know it sounds like an infomercial but exercise will increase your lung capacity and the exchange of oxygen and carbon dioxide as well. This aids in the elimination of metabolic and toxic waste. It helps to keep your bowels moving so you don't get constipated, further reducing the buildup of toxins in the body. Toxic burden and inflammation are known factors contributing to cancer (Weil, 187-193). Exercise will help build and maintain your muscle mass and increase your strength and flexibility. So as the saying goes, "move it or lose it." What you lose may be your life.

This does not mean you have to be a fanatic when it comes to exercise. Find a balance. Everyone can exercise even if it means sitting in a chair and doing arm and leg raises.

You may now be wondering how much exercise is necessary to get the overall benefits. The general recommendation is to do some form of aerobic activity five-to-six days per week for a minimum of thirty minutes. However, for weight loss you are going to want to get up to forty-five-to-fifty minutes. You don't have to do this all in one session. You can break it up into two or three smaller session if you would like. If you are new to a regular exercise program, start out slow or you will just get frustrated and won't stay with it.

Does this mean you have to go jogging? No. Do you have to spend money on a gym membership and buy attractive workout clothing? No. Exercise is not meant to be a fashion statement. It is a health statement. The first thing you want to decide is what kind of activities you think you would enjoy doing. If there is a game you like to play such as basketball, skating, or tennis then go for it. Make it fun, not work. Are you the type that would be more committed in an exercise class or working out in the privacy of your own home? If you are working out in your home, get an exercise DVD that appeals to you. They are inexpensive and it is like having your own personal trainer in the privacy of your own home.

When doing aerobic activity you want to try and get your heart rate up to 60-80% your maximum heart rate. This can be calculated by subtracting your age from 220. Then multiply this number by the 60-80%. Start at the lower percentage if you have more health risks such as obesity, cardiac or pulmonary conditions.

For example, if you are 60 years old are overweight and you have a history of heart disease you calculate your maximum heart rate as: 220-60 = 160 x .60 = 96. If you are already a very health 60 year old and have no risk factors your maximum heart rate would be: 220-60 = 160 x .80 = 128 (Musnick, 481-487).

Before you begin any exercise program it is always a good idea to be evaluated by your health care provider. If you have not had a complete physical in the last few years, now would be the time to get it done. There is nothing more frustrating than to have all good intentions of beginning an exercise program to only be sidelined by an injury or worse, having an undiagnosed heart condition.

Once you are ready, start out slow and gradually increase the time and intensity of your exercise program. A good exercise program should combine aerobic activity with strength training and flexibility. Stated another way: walk, lift weights, and stretch. You don't have to do all of these in the same session. Walking is a very cheap way to exercise. You just want to have a good pair of shoes. Weight lifting can be achieved with a pair of cheap weights, resistance bands, a pair of canned foods, or your own body weight as resistance. For stretching you want to wear comfortable loose-fitting clothing.

None of these are expensive. So if your excuse is that it costs too much to exercise, I think you just lost that argument. You certainly can spend thousands of dollars on gym memberships, exercise equipment, and fancy clothing if you want but it isn't necessary to get into better shape and improve your health and well-being.

One of the best ways to make efficient use of your time is to find an exercise activity that combines at least two, if not all three aspects of a good exercise program. As mentioned, these are aerobic, strength, and flexibility. A good example of this would be yoga or Pilates, which combine the strength and flexibility aspect. There are many different forms of yoga. Probably the most common form practiced is Hatha yoga that focuses on stretching and strengthening various muscle groups (Smith, Greer, Sheets, Watson, 22-29). Pilates, developed by Joseph Pilates, was designed initially to help wounded World War I veterans, who were partially immobilized to gain strength, and flexibility of core muscle groups.

Both forms of exercise are ultimately meant to achieve the same goal (Wood). You can then add a brisk walk to this routine to get the aerobic aspect in order to make your exercise program complete. This is just one example. The idea is to find a combination of activities that addresses the three key areas mentioned.

You might be thinking there is no time in my day to fit in all of this activity. Let's look at it another way. How do you feel now without exercise? Are you tired, having trouble sleeping, depressed, stressed, and overweight? This does not make for a very enjoyable quality of life. Most women I know, and I'm sure some men, always put everyone else first and themselves last.

Does this sound familiar? I am asking you to make an appointment with yourself. Just tell your family and friends that you have an appointment. I am not unlike the rest of you. I live a very busy life. I am married and have two daughters and for this I am grateful. While I was in graduate school, I was still working full-time and raising a family. I still made an appointment with myself everyday to exercise. This helped me sleep, cope with the day to day stressors, and keep my mood stable.

Some of you might be stressed at the thought of exercising. If you keep with it for at least three months, it is likely to become a habit. It will be stressful to some at first, but the longer you commit to making exercise a part of your life, your perspective likely will shift from feeling stressed at the thought of exercise to feeling stressed if you don't exercise. Some of you may not buy this. I encourage you to stick with some form of exercise as there are enormous health benefits. Most importantly, don't try and compare what you are doing with someone else. The only one you are competing with is yourself. Don't try and go out and bench press two-hundred pounds like the man next to you. You can get good results with five-to-ten pound weights. Design an exercise program that is right for you.

One word of caution with any exercise program, moderation is key. Just like any other area in life if you do something too little or too much you will not reap the benefits. Exercise is no different. As John Abdo stated so well in the April 1998 issue of *Life Extension* magazine,"I believe many athletes might actually be shortening their life spans with the intensity at which they train. The loads they subject themselves to during training often overburden their bodies. The frequency of training sessions, recuperation time between workouts often is not adequate enough to repair the damage from previous workouts. The athlete who is constantly training beyond his or her metabolic capabilities is subject to a variety of ailments, including tissue damage, hormonal imbalances, immune system dysfunction and depression. Combined with the vast array of performance-enhancing drugs, such as anabolic steroids and amphetamines, some athletes are destroying their health while striving for gold medals. In addition, the athletes who live long, productive lives after retiring from their sports are those who have paced their training in direct parallel with their metabolic capabilities" (Abdo). You want to pace your routine to your abilities without overextending yourself.

Take Away Tips

- Start moving and be consistent.
- Strive to exercise five-to-six days per week for thirty-to-fifty minutes.
- Combine all aspects of a healthy exercise program: aerobic, strengthening, and flexibility.
- Don't beat yourself up, just keep trying and pace your activity.
- Have fun. Find activities you enjoy.

CHAPTER FIVE
Diet

What is the dreaded four letter word many people despise and would rather not face? You guessed it: diet. I know what you must be thinking here. I have tried so many diets and none of them work. Sure, I might lose some weight, but I always gain it back. I don't like to be told I can't eat something. When I am stressed I eat. My family is not going to eat a bunch of vegetables and so I end up fixing something everyone will eat. I know I am eating too much but I can't stop myself. I like chips and cookies too much. I can't fix one meal for me and a different meal for my family. It is too expensive to eat healthy. I don't have time to eat healthy.

There is that time thing again. Should I go on? What is your health worth to you? Would you rather find out some day you have high blood pressure and diabetes and start taking drugs that are expensive to manage these conditions? Even worse, what is the cost of all those medical visits, hospitalizations, and surgeries due to the complications? I don't mean to scare you, but it is important to realize there are real health consequences related to a poor diet. A poor diet is not unlike smoking. Instead of ingesting cigarette smoke, you may be ingesting foods that are increasing the toxic body burden with poor food choices. These poor food choices can increase your risk of disease and disability.

I am not going to ask you to go on a diet. We all know that they are only a temporary fix to a bigger problem. Unless you are willing to make permanent changes to your standard diet, your struggle with weight and your health risks will always be greater than the person that has made a conscious decision to change the way they look at food and the food choices they make.

Food is meant to provide the body with nutrition and to be a pleasurable experience as well. There is no joy in the thought of depriving yourself. However the reality is that unless you change your perspective on what are enjoyable foods, you will continue to feel deprived. This is whether or not you are on a so-called diet. I am going to ask you to look at the word diet another way with the following acronym. **Do I Eat This?** Do I eat this piece of pie? If, I don't eat this piece of pie, what is a healthier alternative? It could be a piece of whole fruit instead. It could also be a piece of pie, but let's make it a piece of pie that is full of natural, whole ingredients. This way you don't have to feel you are being deprived.

Have you ever spent a day avoiding the so called forbidden food to only give in by the end of the day? Instead of just getting it over with and having a piece of pie, you end up eating the whole pie. I don't want you to have to feel this way. Changing your relationship with food is not just about the food, but it is often an emotional experience as well. Like the person trying to quit smoking, if you go cold turkey, your chances of long-term success are very small. Sure some people have been able to stop smoking this way, but more often than not, many more people will not be successful taking this approach. The same can be said when attempting to change your diet.

If you go cold turkey from eating a poor diet and move a hundred percent to eating organic raw fruits and vegetables how long do you think you will last? My guess is not very long. A better approach would be to keep nudging yourself in the right direction of eating a healthy and nutritionally balanced diet. The ultimate goal is to consume a diet rich in fresh whole organic foods.

So what are healthy food choices and where do you begin? There are many opinions and books written on the subject. I am sure you have read some of them. Very simply, you want to eat foods that are close to the earth. In other words, eat as many foods as you can in their natural form. Ideally you want these foods to be organic when it comes to grains, nuts, fruits, herbs, and vegetables. You want your meat and dairy to come from grass-fed and hormone free animals. If you do buy something that comes in a can, box, or bottle, make sure you can identify and pronounce all of the ingredients on the label. On your trip to the market, try to shop mostly in the outside isles. That is where you will find most of these products.

When you are trying to figure out how to prepare these whole foods, I would recommend buying a Mediterranean cookbook. I do feel the Mediterranean diet is probably the healthiest way to eat. This diet is based on a way of life of people living in countries around the Mediterranean Sea. It is a social experience. The Mediterranean diet consists mainly of extra virgin olive oil, whole grains, nuts and seeds, fresh or dried fruit and vegetables, fish, a moderate amount of dairy and meat, flavorful spices, and wine (United Nations Educational, Scientific and Cultural Organization). This way of eating places an emphasis on several keys factors. To not sound like a broken record, you want to consume plant-based foods such as whole grains, legumes, nuts, vegetables, and fruit. You want to use healthier fats such as olive oil, cold pressed virgin rice oil, and even cold pressed extra-virgin coconut oil.

To enhance the flavors of foods, use lots of fresh herbs and spices. Consume fish and poultry at least twice a week and limit red meat to a couple of times a month. Drinking red wine in moderation is optional.

There is a strong body of evidence that shows that if you consume a Mediterranean diet you are significantly decreasing your risks of most chronic diseases. According to a report from the Mayo Clinic, an analysis of one-and-a-half million healthy adults who followed a Mediterranean diet reduced their overall risk of cardiovascular disease, cancer, Parkinson's and Alzheimer's disease. This is why so many scientific organizations strongly encourage people to make a change in their eating to a more Mediterranean flare (Mayo Clinic).

The *Journal of the American College of Cardiology* published a meta-analysis in 2011 analyzing the results of fifty studies involving 535,000 people and the effects of a Mediterranean diet on metabolic syndrome. The report showed that a Mediterranean diet helps lower blood sugars, triglycerides and blood pressure (Kastorini, et.al, 1299-1313). What this means is that you can lower your risk of developing diabetes and if you already have diabetes you can improve your control of the disease and decrease your risks of developing further complications of the disease.

There was another study done on a group of people after having their first heart attack. They were asked to follow a Mediterranean type diet that included an increase in vitamin-C-rich fruits by twenty percent The study, known as the Lyon Diet Heart Study, showed an astounding seventy percent decrease in all cause mortality (death) or heart disease complications (de Lorgeril et.al., 779-785)!

I would guess that most of you reading this book have been personally impacted by either one or more of the diseases mentioned here. I know I have. My own father died at sixty-four from a heart attack. He had open heart surgery to replace four clogged coronary arteries when he was fifty-one. Almost all of his nine brothers and sisters died prematurely and suddenly from various cardiovascular diseases. My mother has diabetes.

Some of you may be saying that these conditions run in your family and there is nothing you can do about it. I have heard it from my patients many times. I do not want to accept that as my fate. I don't think you should either. Does genetics play a role in your health? Sure. However, it is only one factor. So many of the things we are discussing throughout this book are even more important than your genetics. Two things that are at the top of the list that can contribute to disease are eating a poor diet and the other one is stress. You have the power to change your own destiny. These are lifestyle factors you have the power to control.

If you think converting to a Mediterranean diet seems a bit overwhelming, I just ask you to start taking steps in that direction. One way that I would recommend doing that is to start picking foods that have a low glycemic index. The glycemic index (GI) is a system of ranking the quality of the carbohydrates in food and how they affect blood sugar. It was developed by the Human Nutrition Unit, School of Molecular Biosciences at the University of Sydney.

Foods with a lower GI have been shown to improve weight control, cholesterol and blood sugars. Foods that have a high GI will cause a spike in blood sugars and be like being on a roller coaster. This creates increase body stress and inflammation. This increased inflammation can then lead to problems with digestion and absorption of nutrients, tax the liver, and contributes to insulin resistance and diabetes. It is also contributing to a national epidemic of fatty liver disease. Fatty liver disease causes scarring of the liver. This scarring can progress to cirrhosis of the liver. Sadly I have seen this in some of my patients in their twenties.

Lower glycemic foods help support a steady rise and fall in blood sugar and this will create less stress on the body's metabolic pathways. You want to try and pick foods that have a glycemic index less than fifty. The glycemic index scale ranges from zero to one-hundred. If you are trying to determine if a food has a high glycemic index you can go to www.glycemicindex.com where you can find the glycemic index for various food items (Glycemic Index).

If you would like to take a more in-depth look at how diet can affect your health, I would encourage you to read *The China Study* by T. Colin Campbell, Ph.D., and his son Thomas Campbell II, M.D. It is a fascinating look at how diet, and in particular, animal-based products contribute to disease. The information they gathered during twenty years was derived from studying the lifestyles of 6,500 rural Chinese. It is probably the best long term study ever done on nutrition and its impact on disease.

The Mediterranean diet allows for animal-based product consumption, the results of the *China Study* do not advocate for consuming animal-based products. I know this is probably where you are starting to feel frustrated and confused. Every day you hear about how something you are eating that you thought was healthy is now unhealthy.

In reality, the Mediterranean diet is very close to what Campbell's findings showed. The Mediterranean diet is mostly a plant-based diet with a touch of animal-based products sprinkled on. If you were to look at a food pyramid of the Mediterranean diet your vegetables and fruits are the foundation holding everything else up and animal products are on the tip or consumed to a much lesser degree. In their book, the Campbell's summarize eight principles of food and health.

1. Nutrition represents the combined activities of countless food substances. The whole is greater than the sum of its parts.
2. Vitamin supplements are not a panacea for good health.
3. There are virtually no nutrients in animal-based foods that are not better provided by plants.
4. Genes do not determine disease on their own. Genes function only by being activated, or expressed, and nutrition plays a critical role in determining which genes, good and bad, are expressed.
5. Nutrition can substantially control the adverse effects of noxious chemicals.
6. The same nutrition that prevents disease in its early stages can also halt or reverse it in its later stages.
7. Nutrition that is truly beneficial for one chronic disease will support health across the board.
8. Good nutrition creates health in all areas of our existence. All parts are interconnected (T. Campbell, Campbell, 225-240).

So how should you start to change your way of eating for life? As I mentioned before, do not think that you have to make this change all at once. Start exploring by trying new foods. Try foods of different ethnicity. For example, if you have never eaten Indian food, go to an Indian restaurant. Learn what kind of ingredients they are cooking with and then try to incorporate some of these into your diet. You also want to try shopping at health food stores, and ethnically diverse grocery stores such as an Asian market. Don't be afraid to ask for help. More and more grocery stores are incorporating a diverse variety of these foods into their stores making them more available. More and more consumers are demanding it as well.

I think we are waking up to how vitally important good nutrition is to our health. If you are having trouble trying to figure out how to cook with your new-found ingredients you can search the Internet for recipes or buy a cookbook. Start by trying a different dish at least once a week. Before you know it you will have changed your entire diet for a diet that is rich in the vitamins and minerals necessary to sustaining a healthy life.

You have a good understanding now how important good nutrition is to preventing and controlling disease. You also know that poor nutrition creates havoc with our health. A poor diet creates inflammation and inflammation leads to the manifestation of a whole host of diseases. Chronic diseases are going to have an estimated forty-seven-trillion global and economic impact over the next twenty years.

Suppose you are following a Mediterranean diet and you are still not seeing the improvement in your weight, blood sugars, blood pressure, or joint pain you had hoped for? What is going on? If you are eating a healthy diet and not seeing the results that you want you may have a food sensitivity that is continuing to fuel the inflammation in your body. Food sensitivity issues are a growing problem. They are very under-recognized considering the impact they can have on your health.

Sadly this problem is not on the radar screen of most health professionals. I am not talking about a food allergy that results in a severe allergic reaction with itching and feeling like you can't breathe. What I am talking about is more subtle. You may have fatigue, headaches, joint pain, high blood pressure, blood sugar problems, joint pain, trouble sleeping, and difficulty losing weight. You may blame these problems on stress or getting older but what if this isn't the reason? What if the reason you feel like "crap" is a food sensitivity you didn't even know you had? It has been said that we may crave the very foods we are sensitive too. The top four food sensitivities are gluten, dairy, soy, and eggs.

There are tests available to check for food sensitivities, your health care provider may not know about. Some tests are more sensitive than others. You can also try a food elimination diet whereby you remove one food group from your diet for one month and see if you don't start feeling better.

If you are lucky to have a health care provider familiar with the health impact related to food sensitivities, you may choose to have testing done. Just be aware that it unfortunately is sometimes difficult to get insurance to pay for these tests. I think it would be in their financial interest to pay for these tests. If you find out you have a food sensitivity that may be contributing to your health issues would you not want to remove it from your diet? Just think how much money could potentially be saved if you only knew this could be one of the root causes of your chronic health problems?

I think more and more of the general public are more aware of food sensitivities than their health care professional may be. It is an issue that is often minimized or not given much credit. Gluten sensitivity in particular appears to be a growing problem. Gluten is a protein found in wheat, rye, barley, oats, and spelt.

Many of the whole grains you are eating with devotion may actually be making you ill. Why is that? Sadly, many foods today contain genetically-modified grains. They are molecularly different from the grains produced fifty or more years ago. For example, today's wheat is much higher in gluten and amylopectin A which is a super starch. That is one of the many reasons why people have become a mess of inflammation and obesity looking for their next carbohydrate fix.

What you don't want to do is go fill your pantry with a lot of gluten-free processed and packaged products. Instead, use grains that do not contain such high gluten content such as rice, quinoa, millet, tapioca, corn, buckwheat, arrowroot, and almond flour (Hyman). We will talk more about how food sensitivities create inflammation when we discuss gastrointestinal inflammation in a later chapter.

You should know what you are eating. Since the advent of genetically-modified foods, better known as GMOs, there as has been a rise in chronic disease. Most of the food that you and your family are eating today has been genetically modified. That is unless you are eating only organic.

At the time of writing this book, California was the first state voting to have food labeling change through Proposition 37. Proposition 37, if it had passed, would have required foods that have been genetically engineered be marked on the food label. This was geared to increase consumer awareness as to how the foods they are eating were grown. Needless to say, many large food manufacturers fought this effort and spent millions to oppose Proposition 37.

Unfortunately Proposition 37 did not pass, but it came very close. It is hoped that someday we as consumers will be fully informed of where our food is coming from. We deserve to know.

Why should you care if your food has been genetically engineered? The reason you should care is because these foods can be affecting your health. There is significant research that backs this up and researchers in the field of environmental medicine are trying to sound the alarm.

Genetically engineered foods were introduced into our food in the last twenty years. Nearly ninety percent of corn, soybeans, and sugar beets are genetically modified. It is estimated that three out of four foods are genetically modified. Many European countries have already banned GMO's, but our own Food and Drug Administration (FDA) states they are not harmful.

In studies where rats, animals, and even humans removed GMO's from their diet, their health improved significantly. Some of the diseases believed to be linked to GMO foods are irritable bowel disease, ulcerative colitis, gastro esophageal reflux disease (GERD), food and environmental allergies, asthma, auto-immune diseases, diabetes, cancer, and elevated cholesterol. Since the introduction of GMO's the incidence of GERD has doubled.

When people are taken off GMO's symptoms improved or went away completely according to Dr. Robin Bernhoft, past president of the Academy of Environmental Medicine. According to Jeffrey Smith, a documentary film producer, the FDA ignored the advice of their own scientist who advised more long-term studies were needed to study the potential health effects of GMO's (Oz). It will likely be impossible to remove GMO's from your diet completely, but reducing your exposure to them may change your health.

So how do you begin to change your relationship with food? Don't skip breakfast. This is probably one of the biggest mistakes people make. You want to eat at least three meals and one to two snacks daily. Another way to look at it is, try to eat something every three to four hours. This will help stimulate your metabolism. It is like throwing a log on a fire. In order for the fire to keep burning it needs fuel. In the case of your body this is your metabolism. Eating stimulates the metabolism and skipping meals slows the metabolism or puts out the fire.

You want to use the right kind of fuel. In this case we are talking about nutritious foods packed with vitamins and minerals.

You basically are having four to six feedings daily. For example, you might start off your day with a vegetable omelet, then mid-morning you have a piece of fruit. For lunch have a spinach salad with fish and then an afternoon snack of a handful of almonds. If you are doing this you are less likely to over eat or over snack on the wrong kinds of foods full of sugar and empty calories. For dinner have a lean chicken breast, salad, and a sweet potato. Use lots of fresh spices and herbs to flavor your food. Be sure to drink plenty of water to flush your system and to stay well hydrated. For dessert have another piece of fruit.

    Wow! Doesn't that sound like a lot of food? These meals are packed with vital nutrition including vitamins, minerals, and amino acids. I know you can do it! If it means starting with one meal, then two, eventually you will get to your goal. You will start feeling better, have more energy, and be clearer thinking as well. You will naturally be decreasing the inflammation and toxins in your body. Don't replace meals with a hand full of supplements and then continue to eat poorly. You will be kidding yourself and will be wasting your money on supplements. You have to change the way you are eating.

    Food is not the enemy, you are. As I mentioned before, eating is an emotional experience. In order to change your relationship with food, figure out what emotion is driving your food choices. You can do this by asking yourself, when you are deciding on whether to eat something or not, how do I feel? Why am I choosing to eat this apple or piece of cake? How am I going to feel after I eat it? Do you eat the wrong things when you are under stress, sad, happy, or angry? When I am stressed I eat…..You fill in the blank. If it's unhealthy, then what can I replace it with the next time and in order to make a healthier choice?

When you go to the market, don't go hungry? You want to plan meals out to some degree ahead of time. Make a list and stick to it. Avoid bringing home your weaknesses such as alcohol, cookies, and chips. If they are not in your home to begin with, the temptation to grab these items during a moment of weakness will be less because you would have to make another trip to the market to get them. Out of sight and out of mind will become more a reality.

A lot of us are chronically dehydrated. In order for your metabolism to create steam for the engine it needs water. You want to drink at least half your weight in ounces daily. So if you weigh a hundred-fifty pounds, you want to drink at least seventy-five ounces of water daily. I have heard many people say they are not thirsty or that drinking water is boring. So they end up drinking coffee or even worse they are drinking sugar-laden beverages such as soda or energy drinks. Diet soda is no better as it has been shown to increase appetite and carbohydrate cravings. Diet sodas are mainly sweetened with artificial sweetener. This is a chemical. Do you really want to be drinking chemicals all day long?

These beverages will not only contribute to inflammation and impede weight loss, but they also will further dehydrate you. If you don't like drinking plain water, drink some herbal teas. Herbal teas come in a wide variety of flavors. You can add lemon to your water, or instead of using ice cubes, put frozen berries in your water. It is delicious! Ideally the water you are drinking should be filtered and be drunk in a glass, not out of a plastic water bottle.

In order to keep your bowels moving and cleansing your system, drinking water definitely helps this process. The other thing that will help keep you regular is fiber. The more processed your food, the less fiber you are consuming. Foods eaten in their natural form, such as your grains, vegetables and fruits are higher in fiber. You want to strive to consume at least thirty grams of fiber-rich foods daily.

Don't eat while you are distracted. How often are you eating while watching television, reading a book, or talking on the phone? Don't get to the point of feeling starved. Doing either of these things leads to unconscious eating. Your awareness of the amount of food you are eating - and sometimes what you are eating- will be unclear.

How often do you have trouble recalling what you ate even at your last meal? Slow down! Eating should be a pleasurable experience that you savor. Do you spend thirty-to-sixty minutes to make a meal to only eat it in less than five minutes? If you eat too fast you will likely overeat. You have not given your brain time to catch up with the signals in your stomach. This takes about twenty minutes.

How many Thanksgiving dinners have you sat down to starved, to only then stuff yourself and feel miserable and bloated? Generally you will hit the wall of misery in about twenty minutes. This is because your stomach has caught up with your brain signals to tell you that your stomach is full. So if you chew your food thoroughly and slow down your eating time there is less chance that you will overeat and you get to enjoy the experience of eating longer without feeling miserable at the end of the meal.

One way to help this mechanism between the brain and the stomach is to have a full glass of water, chicken broth or a light salad fifteen minutes before you have your meal. Sit down to eat without the television on, or any other distraction. Try to concentrate on enjoying the meal. You likely will feel more satisfied and actually remember what you ate.

To make sure the food portions you are eating are not too large, try using a salad plate instead of a large dinner plate. Make sure your plate is full of colorful foods, *not* white foods. White foods are generally highly processed and stripped of vital nutrients. If you are full, stop. Don't feel like you have to eat everything on your plate. I know it is that childhood guilt creeping in of how your parents told you there are starving people in the world and you need to clean your plate. Stop the guilt! It could be sabotaging your weight loss. Donate to your local food pantry instead. When you donate to the local food pantry, be sure to provide healthy fruits, vegetable and whole grains. The families that rely on food pantries need to eat healthy too.

Everybody likes to go out to eat at a nice restaurant once in a while. This can quickly sabotage your efforts to eat healthy. Have a plan before you go out to eat. Many restaurants now post their nutritional information online and through downloadable phone applications for tech-savvy readers.

You can look at their menu before you go out to the restaurant and select healthier options. You may save yourself from picking something that has an entire day's worth of fat and calories for something more appropriate. Restaurants often serve food portions that are too large as well. Instead of being one serving you may actually have a plate of food that contains two to three or even four servings. Always aim to eat half and take the other half of your food home for another meal. It is like getting two meals for the price of one every time you go out to eat.

You can also ask how a food is prepared. You want to stay clear of foods that are fried, coated, or creamed. Strive for food choices that are baked, steamed, broiled, or raw (fruits and vegetables). Have your salad dressing on the side so that you can control the amount of dressing being used. One trick here is to dip your fork in the dressing and then pick up the salad on the fork. You will naturally consume much less dressing. Vinegar-based dressings are your best bet but if you do use a creamy dressing, using the fork-first approach should help decrease the number of fats and calories you are consuming.

If you are going to a party, bring the vegetable tray, not the casserole.

Common sense tells us that eating whole grains, fruits, and vegetables is good for us, but what about fats? Not all fats are bad. We have all become more aware of how bad trans-fatty acids are and the inflammation havoc they play. Many of the foods you eat now proudly display "no trans-fatty acids" on their food labels. Including that margarine spread you are using. Like other food sources, fats are best if used in their natural form, and also if they contain more monounsaturated fats as compared to saturated or polyunsaturated fats.

Saturated fats are harder for our body to break down and are solid at room temperature. Animal products contain saturated fat and cholesterol. You want to limit the amount of saturated fat you consume from animal sources. This is an issue for many people. As far as cholesterol is concerned, our bodies do need a small amount of extra cholesterol in our diet, the rest our own bodies produce. The liver actually makes cholesterol and in the right amount helps in the production of vital hormones our body needs.

An egg is a complete protein, meaning it contains amino acids. There is a lot of dispute on whether or not we should eat eggs. Egg whites do not contain cholesterol. I think an occasional free range organic egg is fine. Polyunsaturated fats are not going to stimulate our liver to make more cholesterol and can be good or bad. They are a bit easier for our body to metabolize than saturated fats and contain healthy Omega-3 fatty acids and are considered cardio protective. They are generally liquid, not solid like the saturated fats. Examples include corn oil, vegetable oil, and the best of the group, extra-virgin olive oil.

Monounsaturated oils are the least complex of the oils for our body to use. They also can be the most unstable and become rancid quicker. Rancid oils will increase the oxidative stress on the body and thus inflammation as well. They generally come from a plant-based source, but can also be found in red meat. Fresh is best here and examples include canola oil, safflower oil, grape seed oil, olives, nuts, and avocados. Your diet preferably should contain more polyunsaturated and monounsaturated fats versus saturated fats.

A word of caution to note here is to not strive to eat a fat-free diet. The body needs a certain amount of good fats. Some of you may feel that by picking fat-free packaged foods you are eating healthy. Sadly, you are not. Food manufacturers are frequently replacing fat with sugar. So fat-free does not mean sugar-free or calorie free. Our brains and nervous system need the good fats to help keep them functioning properly.

On a Mediterranean diet you would want to consume approximately twenty-five-to-thirty percent of your calories from fat. Of this only seven-to-eight percent would be saturated fat. These good fats would be obtained from fish, chicken, eggs, olive oil, nuts, and (sometimes) red meats (Oldways Preservation Trust).

My general recommendation would be to select butter over margarine because it is less processed and in a more natural form. I would however, limit the use of butter. You are better off using good fats such as flaxseed oil, walnut oil, organic cold-pressed extra virgin coconut oil, extra virgin olive oil, avocados, and nuts.

As mentioned, we all need a certain amount of fats in our diet as they increase satiety, fuel our brains and help moisturize and hydrate our skin. One thing you may have noticed is that I included extra virgin coconut oil. This is considered a saturated fat. It is the safest oil to cook with at high temperatures. The other oils become unstable at higher temperatures and become more harmful. The coconut oil can be used in place of butter or margarine in cooking. You must use the cold-pressed extra virgin coconut oil. Coconut oil that is stripped and produced through dry processing becomes a trans-fatty acid and this is harmful. This is where coconut oil has received a bad reputation. Coconut oil that is cold pressed is reported to have many health benefits. Virgin coconut oil contains medium chain fatty acids (MCFA) known as lauric acid. This is the same fatty acid found in mother's breast milk. I don't think anyone can argue the benefits of breast milk.

The majority of all other fatty acids are long chain fatty acids (LCFA). What makes MCFA so special? The MCFA is smaller in size than LCFA and makes it easier for our bodies to use. The MCFA does not require special proteins or enzymes to penetrate the cell membrane to be used, where LCFA do. This creates less strain on the digestive tract and the liver. It is a readily available source of energy. Organic cold-pressed extra virgin coconut oil has a very long shelf life, up to two years. Almost all other oils we have discussed should be purchased in small amounts because they have a much shorter shelf life.

Before purchasing coconut oil you want to be sure and look for certain things. As mentioned, it should be organic, cold-pressed extra virgin coconut oil that has not been bleached, genetically modified, is made from fresh coconut and not dried coconut or copra, is made without heat processing, and has no chemical additives such as harmful hexane.

There is actually quite a lot of good research on the reported health benefits of coconut oil. Virgin coconut oil can be used both internally and externally. It is not just used in cooking, but has several reported medicinal benefits including enhancing the absorption of many vitamins and minerals. There is research that shows that this purer form of coconut oil can improve energy level, support thyroid function, aid in weight loss, enhance immune function, improve skin, and promote heart health.

In Samoa coconut oil is used as a sun screen and moisturizer. There are published studies that show that coconut oil has natural antibacterial, antiviral, antifungal, and antiprotozoal properties. This is due to monolaurin which can break through the lipid cell membranes of these organisms. There are many more reported medicinal benefits reported, some antidotal and some with strong research backing. If you would like to read more about coconut oil I would recommend you read *Coconut Cures* by Dr. Bruce Fife (6-56).

Sadly we have a national epidemic of obesity in this country and we are also malnourished. Our grandparents had less, but ate better. We are not consuming anywhere near the recommended daily allowance of fruits and vegetables in this country and are consuming too many sugars. We need to get back to the basics of good whole organic foods that are packed with vitamins and minerals. There have been numerous studies done that show how much better organically-grown fruits and vegetables are nutritionally as compared to conventionally grown fruits and vegetables.

At the time of harvest, organic grains, vegetables, and fruits had a significantly greater amount of polyphenols and antioxidants as compared to conventionally-grown and genetically-modified products (Benbrook et. al.,).

It is all about supply and demand. If more of us are buying organic, this will help drive the producers to grow organic. You can see this change happening in your local supermarket. Ten years ago it would be hard to find organic produce. Today more and more of your local markets give you some organic options. We still have a long way to go, but public awareness has caught on and hopefully we will see the organic market continue to grow. Fresh organic and non-GMO foods are best when it comes to healthy eating.

Take Away Tips

- Change your relationship with food.
- Eat organic.
- Follow a Mediterranean diet.
- Choose foods with a low glycemic index of less than fifty.
- Don't replace bad eating habits with vitamin supplements. Supplements are an adjunct to and not a replacement for a healthy diet.
- Good nutrition is at the core of disease prevention.
- Food sensitivities may be affecting your health and ability to lose weight.
- Don't skip meals and eat something every three to four hours.
- Emotions affect eating habits.
- Eliminate processed foods and artificial sweeteners.
- Drink filtered water that is equal to half your weight in ounces daily.
- Consume at least thirty grams of fiber daily.
- Don't eat while distracted by other things like TV or talking on the phone, and *slow down when you eat!*
- At least twenty-five-to-thirty percent of calories consumed daily should come from healthy fats.

- If you fall, just don't lie there. Pick yourself and get back on track with your very next bite of food. Don't wait until Monday. That excuse will not lead to long- lasting changes that will improve your nutrition.

CHAPTER SIX

Supplements

As I mentioned in the previous chapter on diet, you do not want to rely on dietary supplements to compensate for poor eating habits. Unfortunately most of us are not going to get all our nutritional needs met through our diet on a daily basis. Even if you do eat well it is difficult to do.

The natural vitamin and mineral content of our food today is far less than it was fifty years ago before over-farming with chemicals and genetically-modified seeds were developed. So what are dietary supplements and why should I or should I not take them? A dietary supplement, according to the Dietary Supplement Health and Education Act (DSHEA) of 1994, is a substance you might add and supplement to your daily food intake. These substances may include vitamins, minerals, foods, botanicals, and amino acids (Jegtvig).

There is a growing use of supplements as more people are actively engaging in their own health and nutrition. According to a report in 2009 by the Dietary Supplement Information Bureau (DSIB); direct consumer sales of supplements in 2007 was an astounding $23.7 billion. The impact of direct to consumer sales has a further ripple effect on the economy with a total economic impact through jobs and manufacturing estimated at $60.7 billion and over 455,782 jobs (DaVanoz, Heath, Dobson)! The supplement industry is a very big business.

There is a great deal of controversy surrounding the industry as well, often brought on by special interest groups such as the pharmaceutical industry and health care organizations. Consumer demand for supplements is growing and will continue to do so with or without the support of their health care providers.

This is a real problem as less than half of the people using supplements actually disclose this information to their health care provider which can put you at risk. The supplements you take can have either a positive or negative effect with other medications or even the food you eat. I know this to be true in my own practice. When asked if a patient takes any supplements the response may be no or just a multi-vitamin as these are widely accepted.

However, once patients know I am an advocate for natural health and supplement usage, they are more apt to open up. Then out comes the list of what they really take. It may be anywhere from a couple of supplements to, in one case, a page and a half. There in lays the danger and the concern. If you, as a patient, feel like you are going to be judged, you are not going to tell your providers what you are doing. It is then impossible for them to give guidance on those supplements and their possible mechanism of action, benefits, and risks.

Health care providers need to be more open and accepting and need to educate themselves on the risks and benefits supplements can provide. Health care is to be a partnership between the patient and the provider working together to optimize health. You may be taking supplements you don't need. On the other hand, you may be deficient in a vitamin or mineral supplements that a health care provider can recommend for you.

Providers such as myself can also educate you on the benefits and dosing just like I would do if prescribing a prescription medication. Anything that you put on your skin or ingest can be seen as medicinal, whether it comes from a prescription medication, over the counter medication, vitamins, herbals, or food. They all have a function and impact on you.

One of the main arguments around the use of supplements is how do we know they are safe? There are inferior products in the supplement industry, just like there are in the pharmaceutical industry. However, more people die every year from prescription medications as compared to dietary supplements. In 2007 there was not one death reported from taking a dietary supplement as compared to 38,371 deaths from taking over the counter and prescription drugs (Paulozzi; Saul).

It therefore is amazing that the supplement industry has been unfairly attacked. It is also argued that there is no oversight or regulation of the supplement industry. This simply is not true. There is oversight, though not as tight as what is seen with the pharmaceutical industry.

The safety, labeling, and enforcement of dietary supplements are overseen by the Center for Food Safety and Applied Nutrition (CFSAN), a branch of the Food and Drug Administration (FDA). Furthermore, in 1994, the Dietary Supplement and Health Education Act (DSHEA) was enacted to set up guidelines in labeling of supplements and to support funding for research.

There are currently three government programs at the National Institutes of Health (NIH) that investigate the use and benefit of dietary supplements. These three agencies also conduct and compile ongoing research in the industry and include the Office of Dietary Supplements (ODS), the National Center for Complementary and Alternative Medicine (NCCAM), and the Office of Cancer Complementary and Alternative Medicine (OCCAM).

Dietary supplement manufacturers are responsible for insuring the safety of their products. If an adverse reaction occurs, the manufacturer is required, according to the Dietary Supplement and Nonprescription Drug Consumer Protection Act of 2006, to report this event to the Secretary of Health and Human Services within fifteen days. You still want to make sure the supplement you are taking is of good quality. Good supplement manufacturers will take the extra step to insure the quality and safety of their products through independent review.

The U.S. Pharmacopeia (USP) Dietary Supplement Verifications Program (DSVP) will evaluate a product a manufacturer has independently submitted to verify that the quality and purity of the ingredients and make sure that those ingredients are of the amount and strength claimed. You want to look for USP on the label of the supplement you are purchasing.

Some other agencies involved in supplement safety are the Natural Products Association Good Manufacturing Practices (GMP) Certification Program, NSF International Dietary Supplements Certification Program, and Consumer Lab. Let's look at the function of these agencies individually.

The Natural Products Association GMP Certification Program inspects and certifies manufacturing facilities. The NSF International Dietary Supplements Certification Program role is to ensure the safety of supplements produced by manufacturers and that the labeling lists the ingredients and their amount. Consumer Lab is a private company that independently and without bias performs blind testing on supplements. The goal of this testing is to verify the potency, purity, and bioavailability of a product. So as you can see, there are significant oversights and safety measures in place within the supplement industry. To help ensure the product you are purchasing is coming from a quality manufacturer there are some general guidelines recommended by the American Pharmacists Association and they include:

- Purchase products that have a seal of quality.
- Check products out through independent evaluators such as Consumer Lab.
- Purchase from reputable companies. You often get what you pay for.
- If an ingredient cannot be clearly identified, you should avoid it.

- If you have not had a positive result with a supplement, you may need to change brands (American Pharmacists Association).

There are many reasons why people are increasing their use of dietary supplements in this country and internationally as well. People are taking a more active role in their health care. With the advent of the Internet you can quickly search any ailment and come up with multiple sites telling you how to treat it. The down side to this can be a delay in seeking medical attention.

As a consumer of health care you want to be heard and provided a more holistic approach to your care. You want to be seen as a person, not as a disease or symptom and you want more than two- to- five minutes of your health care provider's time. Many of you are concerned about the safety and financial burden of prescription medications. This leads many people to looking for alternatives, often unfortunately without the guidance of a health care practitioner.

Supplements, like pharmaceuticals, have risks and benefits. Risks to consider with supplements may include drug-to-supplement interactions and contraindications, side effects, lack of monitoring, out of pocket costs, and a delay in seeking treatment (National Center for Complimentary and Alternative Medicine).

Some of the benefits of taking supplements are that you are taking a more active role in your health care, supplements are generally safe and have less side effects, there is greater satisfaction that you are doing something for your health, and supplement use generally encourages you to also improve your overall nutrition (Life Extension Foundation, Shumway et.al.).

People choose to take supplements for a many reasons. Often they are looking for relief from a chronic health condition. Some of the most common conditions people use supplements for, either alone or in addition to prescription medications, are diabetes, high cholesterol, arthritis, insomnia, depression, anxiety, high blood pressure, heartburn, menopausal symptoms, enlarged prostate, osteoporosis, and the common cold.

Supplements include, but are not limited to, vitamins, minerals, amino acids, herbals, meal and nutritional supplements, essential oils, and homeopathy. When considering a supplement you want to first determine its purpose. Are you taking it to replace something, such as a meal? Are you adding it to your daily nutrition because you are not getting enough vitamins and minerals in the foods you eat? Maybe you are taking a supplement to help treat an acute or chronic illness. Whatever the reason, it is important to know the function and benefit of the supplement you are considering. There isn't room here to discuss all the options available as they number into the thousands. However, we will take a brief look at some of the options available.

Vitamins

Our bodies need vitamins in very small amounts and are present in our food. Vitamins are very important to our biochemical functioning to keep us well and free of disease.

Vitamins are classified as either water-soluble (B and C vitamins) or fat-soluble (vitamins A, D, E, and K). If you take in more water-soluble vitamins than your body needs, your body will eliminate it naturally. Fat-soluble vitamins however, can attach to your fat cells and when taken in too high a dose can lead to toxicity. You need to know a dose that is safe to take just like you would if you were taking a prescription or non-prescription medication. Vitamins can come in synthetic and natural forms. I would recommend the natural whole food or veggie forms whenever possible as they are derived from food sources.

In brief, each vitamin has a specific function and all vitamins can have an additive affect on your overall health. The *National Institutes of Health* has identified thirteen essential vitamins and their reported functions as follows:

Water Soluble Vitamins

- Vitamin B1 (Thiamine) helps the body cells change carbohydrates to energy. Getting plenty of carbohydrates is very important during pregnancy and breast-feeding. It is also essential for heart function and healthy nerve cells.
- Vitamin B2 (Riboflavin) works with the other B vitamins. It is important for body growth and the production of red blood cells.
- Vitamin B3 (Niacin) helps maintain healthy skin and nerves. It also has cholesterol-lowering effects.

- Vitamin B5 (Pantothenic acid) is essential for the metabolism of food. It also plays a role in the production of hormones and cholesterol.
- Vitamin B6 (Pyridoxine) helps form red blood cells and maintains brain function. This vitamin also plays an important role in the proteins that are part of many chemical reactions in the body. Eating larger amounts of protein may reduce vitamin B6 levels in the body.
- Vitamin B7 (Biotin) is essential for the metabolism of proteins and carbohydrates, and in the production of hormones and cholesterol. It is also good for hair growth.
- Vitamin B9 (Folate) works with vitamin B12 to help form red blood cells. It is needed for the production of DNA, which controls tissue growth and cell function. Any woman who is pregnant should be sure to get enough folate. Low levels of folate are linked to birth defects such as spina bifida. Many foods are now fortified with folic acid (synthetic form). Folate is the natural and preferred form.
- Vitamin B12, like the other B vitamins, is important for metabolism. It also helps form red blood cells and maintains the central nervous system.

- Vitamin C, also called ascorbic acid, is an antioxidant that promotes healthy teeth and gums. It helps the body absorb iron and maintain healthy tissue. It also promotes wound healing.

Fat-Soluble Vitamins

- Vitamin A is helpful for the formation and maintenance of healthy teeth, bones, soft tissue, mucus membranes, and skin.
- Vitamin D is also known as the "sunshine vitamin," since it is made by the body after being in the sun. Ten to fifteen minutes of sunshine three times a week is enough to produce the body's requirement of vitamin D. People who do not live in sunny places may not make enough vitamin D. It is very difficult to get enough vitamin D from food sources alone. Vitamin D helps the body absorb calcium, which you need for the normal development and maintenance of healthy teeth and bones. It also helps maintain proper blood levels of calcium and phosphorus.
- Vitamin E is an antioxidant also known as tocopherol. It plays a role in the formation of red blood cells and helps the body use vitamin K.

- Vitamin K is not listed among the essential vitamins, but without it blood would not stick together (coagulate). Some studies suggest that it is important for promoting bone health. There are different forms of vitamin K and each form has a specific function (National Institutes of Health).

All these vitamins are important and likely easily obtainable through a healthy diet and taking a good multivitamin. However, I would like to touch further on vitamin D. It is very likely you are not getting enough Vitamin D. There seems to be a national epidemic of Vitamin D deficiency. There are many possible reasons as to why this is including poor nutritional intake and lack of sun exposure.

There is debate as to how much supplemental vitamin D one should take as well. Many of your multivitamin supplements have 400 international units (iu) to 600 iu. This is very inadequate for most of us. I would recommend getting your vitamin D level tested. Your health care provider can then recommend a safe dose for you to take. If this is not possible, then you would be safe to take at least 1,000 iu of supplemental vitamin D_3 daily.

Why all the hype over vitamin D? As it turns out, vitamin D is a pro-hormone that can affect thousands of genes and how our cells function. There have been thousands of compelling studies supporting the far reaching benefits of vitamin D. Vitamin D has been shown to help in the treatment and prevention of multiple sclerosis, fibromyalgia, diabetes, arthritis, osteoporosis, psoriasis, heart disease, immune function, obesity, depression, joint and muscle pain, dementia, and hypertension (Holick, 52-57). Therefore, I would recommend taking a vitamin D_3 supplement unless otherwise contraindicated for an underlying health condition. It is always best to discuss taking supplements with your health care provider.

Minerals

Minerals are also very important to bio-chemical functioning, and include sodium, potassium, copper, iodine, selenium, chromium, zinc and several others. Ideally you will get all the minerals you need from your diet and taking a good multivitamin. Some of you may need extra mineral support for a given deficiency or condition. Mineral deficiencies can cause havoc to your health just as a vitamin deficiency can. Let's look at the function some of these minerals perform. Please note that we will only be reviewing a small portion of the more than fifty minerals our bodies need every day. Certain health conditions may require more or less of a given mineral. For instance, alpha lipoic acid is good for blood sugar regulation and liver function. This is one you may not be familiar with. We will be touching on some of the more common minerals here. They include the following:

- Sodium is important to smooth muscle and cardiac function just like potassium. The two together keep our brains and muscles in motion. Sodium is important for blood pressure control and blood volume.

- Potassium plays a very important role in cardiac and smooth muscle contractions, regulation of blood pressure, and nerve impulses.
- Copper is a trace mineral and aids in the absorption of iron. It is important to the production of adenosine triphosphate (ATP), the cell's fuel. It also aids in collagen formation and hormone function.
- Iodine is another trace mineral and is very important to thyroid function.
- Selenium is also important to thyroid function as well as immune function. There's research that shows it may help in cancer prevention by stimulating glutathione peroxidase, a powerful antioxidant.
- Zinc is involved in many biological functions including metabolism of proteins and nucleic acid, gene regulation, energy production, works against oxidative stress that can lead to disease, growth and development, night vision, insulin storage and release, reproduction, immune defense, and more (Vitamin Information Site).

I would like to give some special attention to calcium. Calcium is the most abundant mineral in the body and is found primarily in bones and teeth. However, calcium is integral to nerve, heart, and muscle function. Calcium requires the presence of several other vitamins and minerals to work properly including vitamin D, vitamin K, magnesium, and phosphorus in particular. You are going to be more prone to calcium deficiency if you are postmenopausal, are getting insufficient amounts of calcium and other minerals in your diet, have a digestive system disorder, kidney disease, parathyroid gland disorders, or take medications that can deplete your calcium.

Calcium deficiency can increase your risk of osteoporosis, heart rhythm problems, high blood pressure, rickets, colon cancer, muscle, and nerve problems. Ideally you should get 1,000mg of supplemental calcium daily through your diet and supplement. Needs may vary slightly with age, sex, and certain medical conditions.

There are many different forms of calcium available and some are absorbed better than others. Calcium citrate is one form that is easily absorbed (Ehrlich). Ideally you don't want to consume anymore than 500mg of calcium at one time. Once you go above this amount the rate of absorption goes down. Ideally your calcium should be taken in conjunction with the other enhancing vitamins and minerals discussed. Too much calcium can be problematic, so don't overdo it. You want to find a balance. Too much calcium can increase your risk of kidney stones, kidney disease, constipation, and affect the absorption of other minerals (Office of dietary Supplements). Don't go overboard on any vitamin or mineral supplement. As I mention before, if you eat a healthy diet and take a really good multivitamin you should be able to meet your daily needs. Exceptions would include certain health conditions, deficiencies, or medications that may require you to get more of some vitamins and minerals and less of others

Essential Fatty Acids

In the last chapter we talked about good and bad fats. Unless you do a pretty good job at eating fish, vegetables, and nuts a couple of times a week you are likely not getting enough omega-3 fatty acids in your diet. Here we are going to talk specifically about the essential fatty acids (EFAs) in fish. You have likely heard that consuming fish or taking fish oil is a good thing. However there is also the concern that consuming too much of certain forms of fish can cause mercury toxicity. This can cause confusion if not properly understood.

Our oceans have become very polluted in the last thirty years with chemicals known in short as DDT, PCBs, PBDEs, arsenic, chlorinated dioxins, pesticides, herbicides, radioactivity, mercury and other toxins. Therefore, over consumption of contaminated fish and fish oils can result in these toxins being passed on to humans.

There are cleaner and safer sources by which you can get omega-3s into your diet without adding additional health risks. Fish is not the only source of EFAs. You can obtain them from plant based sources as well, including chia seeds, hemp seeds, flax seed, and walnuts. Marine life based choices are less apt to have absorbed pollutants including microalgae, aphanizomenon flos-aquae (AFA) algae, and marine phytoplankton. Microalgae oil contains two-hundred-fifty percent more docosahexaenoic acid (DHA) than the average fish oil. In fact it provides an optimal balance of DHA and eicosapentaenoic acid (EPA).

These alternative sources to traditional fish oil tablets are not only less contaminated by pollutants but are also less prone to oxidation and the release of free radicals. Free radicals can increase the risk of atherosclerosis or heart disease. Try to incorporate more plant-based EFA options into your diet. Some fish are still considered safe to consume, including wild salmon, northeastern shrimp and Albacore tuna, and tilapia (Clement; Fisher).

So if you can't get one or more of these sources into your diet what type of fish oil is safest? Krill oil is generally considered the better choice as it is less likely to have contaminates. Krill oil is derived from shrimp crustaceans that live at the bottom of the ocean. Krill oil contains phospholipids and is high in eicosapentaenoic acid (EPA) and docosahexaenoic acid (DHA). This makes it easier for our body's to use. The main phospholipid in krill is phosphatidyl-choline that is very important to a healthy functioning nervous system.

There is significant research regarding the benefits of omega-3 fatty acids. Some of the reported benefits are not limited to the nervous system, but also the cardiovascular and musculoskeletal systems as well. Skin, hair and nails, immune system, increased insulin sensitivity, mood, and hormones also benefit from adequate omega-3 fatty acids (Mercola).

There are so many studies reporting multiple benefits, that like vitamin D, this is one supplement that I would certainly consider. In order to enjoy those benefits you absolutely want to make sure you are buying a high quality product and take at least 1,000 to 3,000mg daily with a ratio of 180mg of EPA to 120mg DHA per 1000mg capsule. So as I have said before, do your research before buying this or any other supplement. There are some precautions to be aware of before taking an omega-3 supplement. If you are allergic to fish or shrimp, take blood thinners, or are going to have surgery; you do not want to take this supplement (Natural Standards).

Probiotics

One supplement that has a lot of emerging scientific research behind it and is important to your overall digestive health is something known as a probiotic. Probiotics are healthy bacteria normally found in the digestive tract and have been found to have a significant impact on health. In fact they outnumber the cells in the body ten-to-one. There are billions of beneficial bacteria in the gut living in the small and large intestine with names such as *Lactobacillus and Bifidobacterium.* Unfortunately, poor diet, environmental factors, stress, food sensitivities, and overuse of antibiotics and other medications such as proton pump inhibitors are disrupting the good bacteria and your digestive tracts microflora balance. Probiotics serve several important functions including balancing immune function, to help form a line of defense against harmful bacteria, aid in the production of B vitamins and vitamin K, reduce gastrointestinal inflammation, promote healthy hormonal and nervous system function, aid in the treatment of digestive diseases such as irritable bowel syndrome, Crohn's and ulcerative colitis, and in colon cancer prevention.

Several studies are coming out showing further far-reaching benefits as probiotics search out and destroy and detoxify the body. Probiotics help to repopulate the gut with good bacteria and aid in nutrient absorption. Probiotics can potentially help with those who suffer from depression and anxiety as well. You are probably wondering how this can be. I thought it was all in my head, not my gut? Believe it or not, ninety-five percent of the body's serotonin, a neurotransmitter that affects mood, is actually produced in the gut. There is an enormous gut-brain connection.

If you are currently suffering from a mood disorder, it is important that you consider what may be going on in your gut. Scientists have observed a correlation between low serotonin and irritable bowel disease, poor gut motility or movement, fluid secretion, and pain (Pick, 35-36).

Furthermore, according to Killian, studies on probiotics have shown benefit in controlling hypertension, cholesterol, insulin sensitivity, non-alcoholic fatty liver disease, decreasing carcinogens, liver detoxification, reducing inflammation, and in promoting immune function.

Selecting a probiotic can be confusing as there are several different varieties available and that contain varying strains and potencies of beneficial bacteria. Common strains include *Acidophilus, Lactobacillus, Saccharomyces boulardii*, and *Bifidobacteria*. Different strains may be used for different reasons. Probably the most studied variety is *Bifidobacteria*.

Bifidobacteria is produced naturally by our intestinal tract. As we age the number of beneficial bacteria begins to decrease due to many of the health risks we encounter over time such as stress, poor nutrition, medications, and the environment. Certain foods promote the formation of good bacteria, such as sauerkraut, kefir, miso, and tempeh. However, as we have discussed, many people are not getting a balanced nutritional diet to promote good intestinal health.

Supplementing with a probiotic can help improve intestinal cell function and prevent dangerous organisms and digestive byproducts from accumulating and promoting disease and inflammation. One strain of *Bifidobacteria* known as BB536 when taken in a dose of two billion colony forming units (CFU's), has been shown to improve immune function in people suffering from allergies, and may reduce the incidence of influenza, pneumonia, *Pseudomonas*, and cardiovascular risk (Killian, 29-39).

There are many strains of probiotics and potencies, so researching before you supplement is imperative. Not all probiotics are equal in their effect and function and dosing will vary depending on the strain and reason for taking the probiotic. For example, if you suffer from Crohn's disease you may want to take up to 450 billion CFU's of *Saccharomyces boulardii* (Mullin, Swift, 149-150). I would not take this high of a dose though without the guidance and recommendation by your health care provider.

  A good strain to take for overall digestive health is one that contains a combination of *Lactobacillus acidophilus, Bifidobacterium bifidum, and Bifidobacterium infantis* in a dose of 5 to 15 billion CFU's (Watson, 60-61). As I mentioned, your health care provider or local pharmacist may be able to help you select a probiotic that is right for your particular needs. I would always recommend taking a probiotic when on an antibiotic. The antibiotic's goal is to kill off bad bacteria but it can kill off beneficial bacteria at the same time and create an imbalance in your beneficial bacteria. The unfortunate consequence of this can then result in common side effects such as nausea, diarrhea, and yeast infections that can occur when taking an antibiotic. Taking a probiotic may prevent or lessen these side effects. Make sure that you take the probiotic on an empty stomach and at least two hours before or after taking an antibiotic.

Botanical and Herbals

Botanical and herbal supplements have been used for thousands of years. Their medicinal properties are written about in the Bible and by Hippocrates, who is considered the father of medicine. Many of the medications today were originally derived from a botanical source. A botanical is plant or component derived from a plant that has been shown to have medicinal properties. An herb is a subset of a botanical (Office of Dietary Supplements). It is estimated that three-quarters of the world's population relies on botanicals or herbals in the form of food, medications, supplements, and in cosmetics. Chinese, Naturopathic, and Ayurvedic medicine all rely heavily on the use of herbal remedies.

Many homeopathic remedies and essential oils are also derived from botanical and herbal sources. It is estimated that twenty-five percent of today's pharmaceuticals originated from a plant source such as chemotherapy agents. Digoxin, a well known medication used in the treatment of atrial fibrillation and congestive heart failure was derived from foxglove. Morphine and codeine, widely used for moderate to severe pain were derived from opium.

Natural botanicals and herbals are widely available as noted above. There are too many options available to list here. Some popular herbals used today include garlic, Echinacea, St. John's wort, melatonin, gingko, and kava kava (Botanicals). Herbal supplements need to be treated with caution, just like any other medication you may take. Many herbals, like drugs, can cause interactions with foods, other drugs, have potential side effects, and should be avoided with certain health conditions.

If you are considering using an herbal supplement you want to take some precautions including knowing the purity and quality of the product as discussed earlier. You want to know and weigh the risks and benefits. You can turn to various resources to assist you such as Consumer Lab, Natural Standards Database, health care practitioners knowledgeable in the use of herbal remedies, and pharmacists.

Though we could discuss many great herbal remedies, there are two herbal remedies that are showing great promise and have a lot of research behind them, they are turmeric and chlorella. Turmeric *(Curcuma longa)* has been shown to have potent anti-inflammatory and antioxidant effects. We know that increase inflammation in the body can lead to disease and one way to prevent disease is to decrease inflammation. Some of the reported benefits of turmeric include its cancer-protective effects, and benefits to many body systems affected by inflammation. This would include the digestive, cardiovascular, immune, and musculoskeletal systems. Turmeric spice can be used in cooking or 450 to 600 milligrams in supplement form (Stengler, 444-446).

Chlorella is often referred to as a super food because it is packed with proteins, vitamins and minerals. There have been literally thousands of studies done on chlorella's health benefits to the immune, digestive, and cardiovascular systems. Chlorella helps to rid your body of toxins by its ability to bind the toxins and rid them from the body. For this reason you want to know where your Chlorella is coming from. You want to know how it was manufactured and grown. Was it exposed to chemicals or acid rain? If so, it will potentially bind these toxins and contaminate the chlorella you are taking in good faith.

Ask the manufacturer for an independent lab report to make sure the level of mercury or other heavy metals contained in the supplement are less than 0.01 parts per million (Rowen).

Essential Oils

Essential oils are another botanical growing in popularity. What are essential oils? According to Essential Oil University, established by Dr. Robert Pappas, "essential oils are the volatile, aromatic oils obtained by steam or hydrodistillation of botanicals. Most essential oils are primarily composed of terpenes and their oxygenated derivatives. Different parts of the plants can be used to obtain essential oils, including the flowers, leaves, seeds, roots, stems, bark, and wood.

Certain cold-pressed oils, such as the oils from various citrus peels, are also considered to be essential oils but these are not to be confused with cold-pressed fixed or carrier oils such as olive, grape seed, coconut etc. which are non-volatile oils composed mainly of fatty acid triglycerides" (Essential Oil University). Essential oils are used for many medicinal purposes and can be applied topically, inhaled, and in some cases ingested.

Though essential oils have been around since the dawn of man, true scientific research in the United States has been lacking. However that is changing. In 1997 Weber University completed research to look at the effects of using essential oils versus Penicillin or Ampicillin in treating two common disease causing organisms, *Escherichia coli,* and *Staphylococcus aureus.*

The essential oils used in this case were supplied by Young Living Essential Oils and included Cinnamon, Oregano, Immupower, and Purification. The essential oils were found to have a superior kill rate in the lab setting as compared to either antibiotic (Allen, 1-8). Another study published, by *BMC Complimentary and Alternative Medicine* in 2006 further supports the anti-bacterial properties of essential oils against both gram-positive and gram-negative bacteria (Prabuseenivasan, Jayakumar, Ignacimuthu, 1-8). *The Journal of Essential Oil Research* published by Taylor & Francis Online would be a good resource to look at the latest scientific research on essential oils.

People use essential oils for various ailments. Some examples where you might see an essential oil used are in treating anxiety, allergies, rashes, infection, joint pain, burns, insect bites, heartburn, nausea, headaches, and as a natural cleaning agent. This list is not inclusive. Probably one of the most widely used essential oils is Lavender. This one oil has been used for about everything you can think of including anxiety, burns, rashes, allergies, cold sores, cuts, and as a deodorant (Young Living Essential Oils). Essential oils are generally considered to be very safe and are certainly worth a try.

Homeopathy

Another supplement form that has been around for hundreds of years is homeopathy. Homeopathy was widely accepted in the early 20th Century in the United States. Many hospitals in fact utilized homeopathic treatments. Homeopathy was developed by Dr. Samuel Hahnemann in the late 18th Century. The word homeopathy was derived from two Greek words, homoios: meaning similar and pathos: meaning suffering. The general principle behind homeopathy is "like cures like." Homeopathy does have scientific research behind it to validate its efficacy as a therapeutic treatment modality. Several studies have confirmed the biological activity of homeopathic medicines (Montagnier, 1732).

The North American Society of Homeopaths has published numerous current and ongoing studies in the field of homeopathy. One example of a recent study showed promise against breast cancer cells. Keep in mind this study was performed in a lab. This in-vitro study showed cytotoxic effects on breast cancer cells with homeopathic dilutions (Frenkel et.al, 395-403). You can go to the North American Society of Homeopathy's at www.homeopathy.org to read various research studies that have been done using homeopathy.

The study of homeopathy is rather complex and true homeopaths spends years learning the art and science of this practice. I regularly recommend homeopathic remedies to my own patients. My family and I have personally benefited from these treatments and found them extremely safe and very effective. I was able to expand my own knowledge about homeopathy through the guidance of Dr. Theresa Dale. Dr. Dale is an internationally-recognized naturopathic doctor and certified clinical nutritionist working tirelessly to help teach practitioners like myself to utilize homeopathic treatments and get to the root of disease and healing.

I have personally seen enormous emotional and physical transformations in people I have treated through what I have learned from Dr. Dale and will be forever grateful.

Homeopathic medicines are micro-dosed natural substances derived from botanical, animal or mineral sources. The medicine is diluted or de-concentrated and then vigorously shaken, traditionally referred to as succussion. This process transforms the original substance into a therapeutically-active medicine.

Homeopathy is a safe and natural method to balance the body and allow the body to heal. Homeopathic remedies used to treat are selected on a very individualized basis and can be selected based on an individual's symptoms, personality, and life experiences. The remedy that most closely matches to a person's set of unique symptoms is known as a simillimum. This is not necessarily always the case though. There are remedies that are more generalized. For example, oscillococcinum is commonly used for more acute illnesses such as the flu.

Incredibly, small amounts of homeopathic substances are needed to aid in healing. The potency will vary depending on what is needed. The potency refers to the strength of a remedy. You will see the potencies referred to for example as, 12X, 6C, 30C, 10M or 6LM. The X potency stays in the body a short period of time and can be used safely for repeat dosing. X potencies are used for first aid, trauma, recovery from injury, preventative dosing, sudden illness, seasonal problems, and general family use. C potencies are used for first aid, seasonal ailments and chronic health concerns. A 200C is in the high range of the C potencies. The M potency is used for specific health problems or constitutional treatment. Very high potencies may stay working in the body for months. High LM potencies are very popular and safe for dealing with children's ailments, sensitive people and emotional issues (Dale).

      Homeopathy has survived years of scathing criticism and yet is prospering. In the U.S. Consumer sales of homeopathic treatments reached $870 million in 2009, growing ten percent over the previous year, according to the Nutrition Business Journal estimates. For example, Oscillococcinum alone, that was mentioned, is sold in sixty countries. Estimated annual retail sales in the U.S. are more than $20 million, according to the manufacturer, Boiron. It ranks 49th out of 318 cold and flu brand products that do more than $1 million in sales. Other popular homeopathic products include arnica gel for bruises and strains and diluted zinc remedies for colds (Deardorff).

      Finally, there is one thing to be aware of when using a homeopathy. There are certain elements that can decrease their effectiveness and should be avoided while using a homeopathic remedy. According to the FDA Homeopathic Pharmacopeia, caffeine, X-rays, perfume, scented lotions, and even essential oils can decrease or negate the effectiveness of the homeopathy (Dale, 188-202).

As you can see there are many different supplements available. Some people will spend hundreds to thousands of dollars every year on supplements. There are many high quality supplements to pick from. Unfortunately there are also many poor quality supplements to pick from. Before buying a supplement, if at all possible work with a trained health practitioner that is knowledgeable in the function, benefits, risks, potential interactions, and dosing of the supplements you are considering taking. This person can likely help you pick out a brand with a reputation for high-quality manufacturing and ingredients. Too often I have seen people of the mindset that if a little is good, a bigger dose would be even better. This is not true. You could be setting yourself up for an undesired reaction or create a biochemical imbalance. Just like Goldilocks in the story of the three bears, you want balance or the dose to be just right. Not too small and not too big. Balance and moderation is the key to everything in life, including supplements.

You should always start with a healthy diet. A natural approach to health is always best, however, a word of caution, do not try to self-diagnose and treat. Unfortunately, I've seen this with less than ideal outcomes. By the same token, those that have come to me desiring a more natural approach to their health can absolutely transform their lives.

Take Away Tips

- Don't rely on supplements to compensate for poor dietary habits.
- Look for USP on the label before you buy.
- Check products out through independent evaluators such as Consumer Lab.
- Purchase from reputable companies. You often get what you pay for.
- If an ingredient cannot be clearly identified, you should avoid it.
- If you have not had a positive result with a supplement, you may need to change brands.
- Take a good quality whole food multivitamin supplement daily.
- Take supplemental Vitamin D3 1,000 iu daily.
- Consume at least 1,000 mg of Calcium daily through diet and supplementation if need. Take in no more than 500 mg at one time. Your diet should contain adequate amounts of magnesium, vitamin D, potassium, and phosphorus to enhance calcium effects.

- Consider taking a probiotic with at least 5 to 15 billion CFU's per dose. Particularly if on an antibiotic or have gastrointestinal disturbances.
- Botanical and herbals may be an option in the treatment and prevention of disease.
- Essential oils have reported medicinal benefits.
- Homeopathy, like botanicals, herbals and essential oils, may be an option in the treatment and prevention of disease and have reported medicinal benefits.

CHAPTER SEVEN
Four undiscovered pathways to health:
Stress, Gastrointestinal Health, Detoxification, and Hormones

We are now going to discuss four key areas that are preventing you from achieving ultimate wellness of the mind, body, and spirit. Suppose you have tackled all of the previous chapters' components one by one and still you are struggling to sleep, lose weight, get rid of joint pain, relieve constipation, your headaches are still not gone, and you are still tired. What is going on? Why don't I feel better? I am eating healthy, exercising, and taking a multivitamin. I have tried improving my sleep and eliminating as many environmental toxins as possible, but I still don't feel as good as I would like.

It is time then to dig deeper. It is time to get to the root cause. You can be doing everything right and be completely unaware of certain aspects that are sabotaging your efforts. So unless those things that are sabotaging your efforts can be identified, your struggle will continue. It is at this point you really need the guidance of a holistic practitioner who is familiar with the assessment, diagnosis and treatment options available to address these specific issues. A trained practitioner can help get to the underlying root cause that is preventing you from nourishing the seeds you have planted up to this point and growing or achieving ultimate health.

What is stopping you from getting the balance you desire of mind, body, and spirit? The block I am talking about here is the role that stress, poor gastrointestinal health, inadequate body detoxification, and hormone imbalance have in hampering your efforts to be at peace in your own skin and the awesome soul you are meant to be. We will break down these four undiscovered pathways to health one by one.

Stress

Who does not have stress in their life? Everyone does. No one goes through life without being affected daily by stress. As mentioned earlier, I believe that stress and poor diet are at the very core of many of the chronic health problems plaguing society today. Using the analogy of the tree, these are the roots that are damaged and preventing you from flourishing. You can't see the roots of a tree, but you know they are there and if they aren't properly nourished the tree will die.

Every human-being has this same problem. If you are not nourishing the roots, you too may wither and die much sooner than you had intended or at least not live a fulfilled life. As we look at stress and its impact on our physical and mental well-being it will also be important to address how integral our emotional health is as well. You cannot talk about stress without discussing how our emotional constitution factors into the mix.

There is a very intimate relationship between stress and emotions and on their impact upon a person's physical, mental, and spiritual balance. If we don't appreciate or accept this very important factor, there will continue to be roadblocks that are consciously or subconsciously placed in our path.

So what is stress? Stress was first defined by Han Selye as the nonspecific response of the body to any demand made upon it and how you perceive a given stressor will determine whether or not you will successfully adapt. This point was further supported by Robert Sapolsky, a professor of biology and neuroscience at Stanford University and his research on the effects of stress. It is not the amount of stress that can affect you as much as your reaction to stress. Sapolsky postulated that stress-related illness could be decreased by having an outlet for your frustration, finding a diversional activity, by having a real or imagined sense of control, and looking for something positive.

According to Oakley Ray, knowledge is power when it comes to how we handle stress. If you were raised to respond to stress in a positive or negative way, you likely are carrying this same responsiveness into adulthood. However, if you learn to adjust your perception of the world around you, stress can be minimized. This can be further supported by a healthy support network along with your spiritual or religious beliefs (Bland, 138-140). To further illustrate this point, studies done by King and Bushwick, showed that ninety-four percent of patients admitted to the hospital believe that spiritual health is as important as physical health. Spirituality and your belief systems have an enormous impact on health and are intimately entwined with the physical response (Liska, 165-166).

How often when you go to your health care provider do you feel that your spiritual and emotional needs are being addressed? My guess is not very often, if at all. In the defense of the hard-working health care providers everywhere, they often are given only fifteen minutes for an appointment. By the time you are checked into the exam room, they may have five minutes left.

Health care is over-regulated and extremely expensive. In order for them to pay the bills, you are run through the system as if you are on an assembly line. This does not foster an environment of healing or the chance for your health care provider to address your spiritual and emotional needs.

This is not only frustrating for you as the patient, but it is also frustrating for many of those health care workers called into what is suppose to be a caring profession. We all need to be present in every way for this experience to be therapeutic. I have seen the impact this can have on you as a patient. It can give you the strength you need to take your life back instead of giving it away.

Let me give you a personal example of how spiritual health impacts stress and healing. Several years ago I received a call that my oldest sister had been rushed to the emergency room and was not expected to live. She was initially given a five percent chance of survival and if she did survive, they said she would likely be in a vegetative state lying in a nursing home the rest of her life.

She was only fifty years old and had just suffered a devastating brain stem aneurysm. Before she was air lifted to the hospital and while on a ventilator, before she lost consciousness, she had the presence of mind to write a note asking for Healing Touch. You see, my sister is a nurse and a Healing Touch practitioner. She also had a strong spiritual and religious belief system in place.

She made it through the first twenty-four hours and was placed in a drug-induced coma. Most people do not survive the first twenty-four hours. All twelve of her brothers and sisters rallied and the Healing Touch community my sister is a part of also came to the hospital to pray.

One healing practitioner came in every day to administer Healing Touch to my sister while she lay in the intensive care unit. During these episodes my sister's vital signs would stabilize or improve. Meditation tapes played very softly in the background. This went on for thirty days as my sister struggled to survive.

A physician who had a reputation of not having the best bedside manner even got in on the action. When one day he walked into the room and saw my sister struggling. He stopped what he was doing to put on one of her meditation CDs for her. Many of us in my family believe that along with the expert medical and nursing staff, if it wasn't for her own belief system and that of her family and friends, she would not be alive today. Yes, after thirty days in the intensive care unit, my sister walked out of the hospital with no long-term side effects. She has been back to work as a nurse helping others for several years now. It was both a horrifying and miraculous experience for all of us.

Why did I share this very intimate story with you? It shows how our perception of stressful events can alter the outcome of health, even against all odds. Whether stress is perceived or real it triggers a physical response in the body. This begins in the brain when a thought is generated. Then that triggers an area known as the hypothalamus which then triggers the pituitary and adrenal glands to respond. This is commonly known as the hypothalamus-pituitary-adrenal axis (HPA-axis).

The HPA axis starts the release of neurochemicals and hormones including cortisol, epinephrine, norepinephrine, inflammatory markers, along with immune-suppressing chemicals. This then alters the release and production of immune protectors and mood stabilizing neurotransmitters. Chronic stress is by far more dangerous than a short-term stressor that resolves quickly. The study of how the mind and body respond to stress is known as psychoneuroimmunology (PNI).

Conscious and subconscious stress has a direct impact on the nervous, endocrine, and immune systems. Nurses understand this concept very well and learn about it very early in their training. That is also why so many nurses like my sister understand the value that meditation, Healing Touch, and various types of relaxation techniques can provide. Holistic providers have a great appreciation for the mind, body, and spirit connection. As a nurse practitioner I have seen amazing expressions of spiritual, emotional, and physical healing that support this principle. The field of PNI supports the notion that stress manifests disease. There are numerous studies showing a correlation between stress and the development of coronary artery disease, cancer, gastrointestinal disorders, memory loss, diabetes, mental illness, autoimmune disease, and even catching the common cold.

Therefore, how one perceives and responds to stress can have either a positive or negative overall impact. In other words, it is not the stress itself that can harm you, but, your reaction to the stressor can. Whoever coined the phrase, what doesn't kill you will make you stronger was probably more right than they knew.

In order to change your perception and reaction to stress you first need to learn how to relax. Learning how to relax can have a profound physiological response. As Herbert Benson, the pioneer of the relaxation response showed, you can go from a human being having a sympathetic nervous system response to a parasympathetic nervous system response (Lorentz, 1-6).

What that means is, going from being on high alert to relaxing by the pool on a warm sunny day. Everything in your very being calms down. Your heart rate and blood pressure come down and you go from being anxious and on edge to a state of calm and peacefulness. You can feel the difference just by creating the thought and feeling how your physical body responds in each of these scenarios.

It is hard to change perception without addressing emotions. A thought or belief can generate twenty different emotions. How you feel emotionally about Monday mornings, may spark a very different emotion in one person to the next. You may be excited about going to work or you may have a feeling of dread. This all depends on your perception and what meaning you give to the situation. It can be very hard for some of you to even tell what emotion you are feeling. So many of us are out of touch with who we are and what we are feeling.

On a conscious level you may feel fine. On a subconscious level you may have repressed emotions and memories that are keeping you from truly feeling and understanding the emotions you may have right now.

If you are unable to take responsibility for your emotional state you may risk staying stuck in thought patterns that can have a negative impact on your health. This is cause and effect. For example, let's say as a child you were told you couldn't do something because you weren't smart enough, pretty enough, clumsy, or maybe you were emotionally, physically, or sexually abused. This in turn creates self-doubt and lowers your self-worth. You embed that thought at a very cellular level and even suppress how you felt when this happened.

Fast forward in time and as an adult you develop fibromyalgia, depression, or knee pain. It is believed those repressed emotions you thought you had put to bed so long ago may actually be impacting your emotional and physical health now as an adult. Does this strike a cord in you? If so, on some level you know this to be true.

Theresa Dale, Ph.D., N.D. put it well when she said, "We must clearly see and feel how our emotions work, instead of being worked over by our emotions and numbing them through dependencies on various substances and activities." It is important to try and identify the trigger that lead to your current beliefs and emotional tendencies. As the Borg, stated in *Star Trek Next Generation,* "resistance is futile."

Dr. Theresa Dale does an excellent job in illustrating how being stuck emotionally can trigger mental and physical upheaval in her book, *Revitalize Your Hormones* (2005). In her book, Dr. Dale applies the principles of Traditional Chinese Medicine's Five Element Theory to unlock the emotion that is contributing to a given health issue.

Keep in mind that this is only one aspect of disease. Disease is the result of multiple factors. According to the Five Elements and emotions, each element of fire, earth, metal, water, and wood has a corresponding set of emotions. These emotions are further impacted by seasons, time of day, sounds, and body organs. Stay with me here. I know this might be a difficult concept to grasp. Let me give you an example. Let's say you have a heart problem. The underlying emotions that you may have suppressed on a subconscious level or have felt chronically could be a contributing factor. Emotions that are connected to the heart are feelings of being overwhelmed, guilt, shock and/or trauma. Let's look at another example. If you have ever dealt with the loss of a loved one, has the grief of that experience been so great that you felt like you couldn't breathe? The organs associated with grief are the lungs. Time of day can also be a clue to identifying where you are stuck emotionally. For example, are you having trouble sleeping at night and find yourself waking up about 2:00 a.m.? You may have conscious or subconscious anger, rage, or frustration to address and if you don't find a way to address it your liver can become overburdened. So if you are out of touch emotionally, this concept may help you to get in touch. If you are in touch with your emotions, this can then help you to alter your perception of those things that are leading to how you respond to real or perceived stressors.

In looking at the specifics of the Five Element Theory and to help you identify if you may have certain emotional blocks, observe how you are feeling during a given time of day. When your energy level is lower this can be a sign of imbalance based on the Five Element Theory. This may be a clue to not only your emotional health, but possibly your physical health as well. How do you feel when you wake up in the morning? Do you wake up alert and ready to start the day or are you struggling every morning to get out of bed and get yourself to work on time? Are you feeling stuck like you don't have the energy to move? The emotion of feeling stuck correlates with low early morning energy. The large intestines or colon is also associated with this emotional block. Have you been plagued with irritable bowel syndrome, chronic constipation issues, or diarrhea? This may be a sign that you feel stuck on some level. Are you in a bad relationship, a job you don't like, or having financial difficulties? This creates additional stress and further perpetuates the problem. Once you get out of bed do you rely on coffee to help wake you up? If this is the case, the underlying emotional blocks connected to this are feelings of despair, depression, and disgust. These may be feelings you have now or may relate to events that happened years ago that you buried in the subconscious and are now having an impact on your emotional or physical well-being. Physically you may be having stomach problems such as heartburn, nausea or eating empty calorie sugar laden foods. You could be feeding a void and while doing so are becoming more tired and stressed.

So you started off the morning with a coffee and donut and by 10:00 a.m. you are really dragging. So what do you do, have another cup of coffee? Maybe you grab a sugary snack thinking that your blood sugar is low and gee maybe a pastry would help perk you up. If you are struggling to get through the morning and self-medicating with coffee, energy drinks, or pastries this can be a sign of blocks in your spleen and pancreas. Emotionally this can be a sign that you are struggling to feel accepted by family, friends, or coworkers. Do you feel like you are not good enough or that everyone is better than you? The underlying emotions of low self-esteem and fear of rejection are emotional blocks present in epidemic proportion. We all want to be accepted for who we are, but often struggle to accept ourselves first. So if you are dragging mid-morning, this may be an area you want to work on and explore further. Another thing to think about here is, look at how many people have diabetes? It is an epidemic? There is a lot of people not feeling good about who they are.

If you don't have problems getting up and starting your day relying on stimulants to get you going you might not have underlying physical or emotional imbalance that correlates with the scenarios presented. The other possibility is they have not presented themselves or you don't have emotional blocks in these areas. Maybe you make it through your morning fine, but you are really tired after lunch. That pizza or sandwich you had for lunch just seems to just sit in your gut or you feel bloated. Your heart feels heavy and you are feeling guilty about eating that pizza instead of the spinach salad you had planned on eating. This can be a sign of imbalance in the heart and small intestine and the emotions of feeling vulnerable, overwhelmed, shock, guilt or repressed trauma. Was there ever a time you felt really vulnerable or guilty and could that be affecting you on some level now. By 4:00 p.m. you are tired and have had it with everyone. Do you feel irritable? Do you get frequent bladder infections or have to urinate frequently? Is there someone who has irritated you at some point and is still bothering you now? Facing this emotion and forgiving may help you to clear this block.

It is now 6:00 p.m. and you are home from work and exhausted and dehydrated because you didn't drink enough water and this stresses your kidneys. Do you fear what life holds for you and your family? Are you afraid of change? Is fear keeping you from progressing? By 8:00 p.m. you are sitting in front of the television set mindlessly watching some program and don't have the strength to read a book, talk to those around you and try to push out thoughts of the day you just had. Sex with your partner becomes a chore instead of a time for a close intimate connection of love and nurturing of one another like it once was. If this is how you feel in the evening the emotional blocks of denial and unresponsiveness can be impacting your sex life. By 10:00 p.m. you are starting to feel anxious about the next day, you have trouble getting to sleep and may rely on anxiety medication or sleeping pills because you feel your life is out of control and your job is stressing you out. This can be a sign of underlying adrenal exhaustion which is affecting your hormone balance, energy level, and ability to adapt to stressors. Your thyroid also may not be functioning at full capacity. Emotionally you might not only feel anxious, but may be suffering from feelings of paranoia and confusion as well.

      Let's say you get to sleep but every night you seem to wake up between midnight and 2:00 a.m. This could be a warning of gall bladder and liver issues. How many people do you know who have had their gall bladder removed? Maybe you have. There is also an epidemic of liver problems in this country. Emotional blocks associated with this period of time are resentment, anger, rage, and frustration. Wow! How much of that have we all seen? You may feel this way towards your family or co-workers. We are all bombarded with negative messages every day that consciously or subconsciously are leading to these emotional blocks in ourselves. Is it any wonder that so many people can't sleep and are reliant on sleeping pills? If you could address those blocks, start sleeping better and get off sleeping pills would you do it? I would guess that you would. By addressing the underlying stressors utilizing different stress reduction techniques you are giving yourself the opportunity to sleep better and to begin to focus on the positives in life, instead of the negatives.

The last emotional block is that of grief. None of us gets through life without suffering this emotion at some point in time. If you find yourself waking up at 4:00 a.m. or have underlying lung problems your grief may be so trapped in your psyche it is paralyzing your lungs. Learn to breath, feel what has caused you grief and face it. Write about it, scream, exercise, or whatever else you need to do to help you release it. Releasing emotional blocks can be a transformational experience. All life's adversities are opportunities for emotional growth and expansion.

In order to help heal these emotional blocks discussed and in continuation with the Five Element Theory you want to look to nature and the elements of fire, earth, metal, water, and wood. These represent the healing properties to help you unlock your emotional blocks. By being fully present and allowing yourself to feel you can find the determination to have balance, joy, and spiritual growth. Nourishing your emotional health can lead to a future full of possibilities and a life of physical, mental, and spiritual abundance (169-177).

You now have a better understanding of how emotions and stress are intimately connected to your mental, physical, and spiritual being. This is an important step. But what happens next? You now own and take responsibility for your emotions and your stress reactions, but how do you now turn them around to work for you and not against you?

Certainly there are plenty of self-help books just like this one out there to guide you. These may give you a place to start. However, you will completely miss the point if you don't learn one very important thing. You must do this for you, not for somebody else. If you are embarking on this endeavor because someone told you to, this may create more negative emotion and further blocks to your healing. You have to desire it for yourself. *Voice what you feel, and feel what you voice.* Don't express what you think others expect or want.

Want only leads to more wanting and you're left spinning your wheels to nowhere. You have to put yourself first. So many of us struggle with this because we don't want to be perceived as being selfish. This is where you need to alter your perception. It is selfish not to put yourself first. I know this seems to go against everything you ever learned. However it is important to realize, if you can't care enough about yourself, how can you adequately care for and nurture others? I would wager a bet that anyone reading this book is guilty of this, including the author. This is something we all struggle with on some level. Please care for yourself and learn to love who you are on every level. This certainly is not done by comparing ourselves to what others are doing. Nor is it achieved by trying to live up to others' expectations of us.

So how do you start taking responsibility for your emotions and stress response? Like Dorothy in the *Wizard of Oz*, just follow the yellow brick road and take one step at a time. This isn't a race, but a path to health and healing.

The path never ends and will have many twists, turns, mountains, and valleys. Just start walking and see where it leads you. Don't allow self-doubt or the negativity of others to put blocks in your path. Just walk around or through the block and keep going. Choose to align yourself with people and places that promote positivity. If you stay around negative energy it will cause you to stray from your path. Instead take a stand to foster gratitude by looking for the positive in every situation (Hirashiki, 36-37).

Let me give you an example. When my husband and I found out the baby I was carrying several years ago was going to be born with a birth defect and that he wouldn't survive, we each dealt with our grief in our own way. Instead of blaming God, I asked Him to help me to survive my grief and carry me through it.

I had two choices, either let my grief consume me for the rest of my life, or look for a positive outlet for it. My son's short life had to have a meaning and purpose. It was at that moment I decided to face one of my fears, which was going to nursing school. I felt I had nothing to lose at that point and I turned my grief into gratitude. I thanked my son for giving me the strength to face my fear. So even in one of the darkest moments in my life, I was searching for something positive to lead me down my own personal path of growth and transformation.

This is not an easy thing to do, but by facing my emotions I was able to foster a feeling of peace and find the determination to change the path I was on.

I did not blame myself, God, or others for what had happened to our precious son. I did not focus on self pity or blame. Instead I learned to be grateful for what my husband and I had, not on what we didn't have. This alone gave us enormous strength to preserve in the face of tragedy. We all have a choice on how we are going to respond to those things that happen to us. Finding gratitude for the little things can help us get through the big things. Gratitude can be a lifeline to hold onto when faced with adversity.

When it comes to stress, there are a number of ways you can help decrease, or in some cases eliminate, your stress level. I would encourage you to try several different methods. Some examples are as follows:

- Write your thoughts and feelings down on paper. No one has to see it but you. Underlying emotions or revelations may be revealed through this process and no one gets hurt. A trained specialist in cognitive behavior therapy can help you learn to change your reaction to stress.

- Say a daily affirmation or prayer to guide you through your day.
- Exercise in the form of walking, yoga, Tai Chi, Qi Gong, or any exercise you enjoy. Don't pick an exercise you dislike if you're doing it to relieve stress.
- Listen to relaxing music.
- Learn how to meditate or listen to recordings in guided imagery.
- Breathe! Slow, deep breathing exercises go a long way to help calm nerves. I usually recommend breathing in through your nose for five seconds, then hold your breath for five seconds, then breathe out through your mouth for five seconds. Try it now. Doesn't it feel great?
- Eat a healthy diet and get adequate sleep.
- Seek out a practitioner trained in energy work such as Reiki, Healing Touch, massage, Quantum Touch or any other relaxation method.
- Other ways of unblocking energy flow and emotions include acupuncture and emotional freedom technique (EFT). EFT involves tapping energy meridians.
- Nurture self-care.

- Engage in a hobby that you enjoy (Mills, Pick, 44-48; Weil, 138-143).

I challenge you to work every day to be in the eye of the hurricane where there is complete peace and calm. Once you go outside the eye of that hurricane, things are spinning out of control with no beginning and no end. When you stay centered, your perception of stress changes and your overall health and well-being improve. The choice is yours to make.

Take Away Tips: Stress

- Stress is a reflection of your belief systems.
- Thoughts create a physiological response. Your stress perception can have either a positive or negative effect.
- Learning how to relax can save your life.
- There is an emotional component to every mental, physical, and spiritual aspect of your life.
- Align yourself with people that encourage positivity.
- Be a survivor, not a victim.
- Stay centered.

Gastrointestinal Health and Detoxification

Have you ever been told that your problem is all in your head? In reality what we should be saying is, "It's all in your gut." Many of the chronic health problems that people are dealing with today are the result of gut inflammation and poor detoxification. Things need to be addressed from the inside out. A healthy gut equals a healthy mind and body. You know that eating a healthy diet is so important. But why is that and what is going on internally that makes this so important? If we are consuming the wrong kinds of food and beverages, are eating too fast and under stress; this will increase inflammation in our digestive tracts and impair digestion, absorption of vital nutrients, and detoxification. Our poor diets and fast paced highly stressful lives are contributing to the national epidemic of chronic health issues such as obesity, irritable bowel syndrome, celiac, Crohn's disease, diabetes, heart disease, cancer, arthritis, headaches, heartburn (gastro esophageal reflux disease), chronic fatigue, fibromyalgia, osteoporosis, nutritional deficiencies, anxiety, depression, and much more.

    The digestive tract starts at the mouth and ends at the anus. But there is a whole lot going on between those two points. As soon as food, or even the thought of food, happens we start salivating and releasing digestive enzymes to aid in food breakdown. Food is then swallowed and travels down the esophagus to the stomach where hydrochloric acid, mucus, more digestive enzymes, and gastrin further aid the breakdown and mixing of foods in the holding tank known as the stomach until things are ready to move on down the digestive tract.

    The door to the next part of the digestive track is then opened. This is the pyloric valve. From here things move on to the duodenum, which is the beginning of the small intestine. Food at this point is known as chyme. Chyme in the duodenum stimulates the release of bile from the liver and gall bladder, bicarbonate, and more digestive enzymes and insulin are released from the pancreas.

Next, things start sliding down through the very long (20-25 feet) and winding road of the small intestine. Within the small intestine there are finger-like projections known as villi. It is across these villi that many important functions happen. Healthy villi in the small intestinal mucosa aid in the absorption of vitamins, minerals, amino acids, and fatty acids. They also aid in the production of healthy gut bacteria and the killing of harmful invading bacteria and parasites.

From here the remaining chyme goes through the next door, the ileocecal valve, into the large intestine. In the large intestine, some the remaining water and nutrients are reabsorbed. What is left is the food waste that is excreted as stool. A healthy digestive tract will produce at least one, but ideally two-to-three bowel movements a day (Watson, 5-13).

I can hear you gasping. Many of you are chronically constipated and are likely saying, "I am lucky if I have one bowel movement every three or four days or maybe longer." This obviously is not healthy and all the waste byproducts you are producing are not being excreted.

A healthy gut equals a healthy life. To understand this further we need to examine the role of three critical defenders or guardians that protect the digestive tract from invasion. The three guardians of the digestive tract are the gastrointestinal flora, mucosal barrier, and gut-associated lymphoid tissue (GALT).

The first of these we will discuss is the gastrointestinal flora, or the balance of beneficial bacteria in the gut. We touched on this earlier in the chapter on supplements when discussing probiotics.

As you may recall, there are billions of beneficial bacteria in the gut living in the small and large intestine. The beneficial bacteria serve several important functions that include balancing immune function, helping form a line of defense against harmful bacteria, aiding in the production of B vitamins and vitamin K, reducing gastrointestinal inflammation, and promoting healthy digestion, along with hormonal and nervous system function.

It is estimated that there are about five hundred varieties of bacteria weighing between five and eight pounds within our intestinal tract. When certain stressors, poor diet, medications, environmental toxins, food allergies or sensitivities, and exposure to harmful organisms come into contact with our digestive tract this creates an imbalance and potential overgrowth of harmful bacteria and yeast.

This compromises the mucosal intestinal lining and leads to the breakdown of this wall of defense.

Bacterial imbalance will increase intestinal permeability or breakdown in the filtration and absorption mechanisms in the gut. This weakens our immune system's ability to fight off the invaders and opens the gates to disease formation and proliferation. This is better known as dysbiosis (Seksik, 44-51). Dysbiosis in the small intestine is associated with several common ailments including chronic diarrhea, rheumatoid arthritis, chronic fatigue, fibromyalgia, hypothyroidism, liver cirrhosis, irritable bowel syndrome, migraine headaches, restless leg syndrome, and rosacea.

Taking a probiotic is one way to help repopulate beneficial bacteria. You can also consume prebiotic-and-probiotic-rich foods such as kefir, kimchi, natto, miso, tempeh, almonds, asparagus, chicory root, endive, garlic, Jerusalem artichoke, kiwi, oats, onions, leafy greens, and leeks. These natural foods help to stimulate the restoration of a healthy gut and reduce intestinal inflammation (Mullin, Swift, 40, 86-89, 148-150).

The next defender protecting our digestive tract is the mucosal barrier. It consists of a layer of epithelial cells, tight junctions, and extrinsic layer. This layer contains a coating of mucus, bacteria, and secretory IgA. Secretory IgA is the guardian defender of the mucosal lining.

The mucosal barrier's job is to police what is allowed to cross back and forth across the intestinal lining. If the mucosal barrier is compromised in some way your body's immune defenses may not be able to keep up with the constant daily attacks presented through your diet, medications, environmental toxins, viruses, bacteria, and the like.

This compromises the host (you) and can open the door to an inflammatory cascade of events to occur. The microvilli in the small intestine become irritated and inflamed thereby wearing down the natural defenses. When this occurs harmful invaders penetrate this wall of defense. Your gastrointestinal tract is now under attack. These invaders can now go after every system in the body (BioHealth). When your defenses are down, so too are IgA levels as well. The wall of defense has now been compromised.

To look at the intestinal or mucosal barrier another way, think of this lining of the gastrointestinal tract as a fort. The fort's job is that of protection from outside enemies. If it comes under an acute attack such as taking a medication short term or a minor stressful event it will likely be able to withstand the attack. However if the fort comes under constant and prolonged attack, holes start to be poked through the walls and your army of defenders weakens.

If the attacks of poor diet, chronic stress, medications, parasites and the like continue your mucosal barrier of protection will become defenseless and disease will likely follow. You may have developed some form of autoimmune disease that is now robbing you of your quality of life. There are many autoimmune diseases that can develop such as lupus, rheumatoid arthritis, hypothyroidism, diabetes, scleroderma, and others.

Your immune system is now completely exposed with no protection. Often times however the symptoms may not be as obvious as these more extreme cases of compromise and will be more subtle. Your fort may be badly damaged but not yet completely exposed. In any circumstance where the fort has been compromised you will find a low IgA level, because it is the guardian of the fort.

Some conditions to which low IgA contribute have obvious consequences as you can see in the analogy given. You know this well if you suffer from any of the health conditions previously mentioned. However, there are many people walking around with less obvious or easily measurable manifestations of low IgA and an impaired digestive tract and malfunctioning intestinal barrier.

You may go years before developing a problem or you may have more subtle and annoying symptoms. Probably the most unrecognized and unappreciated of these are food sensitivities. How many of you have experienced gas, bloating, anxiety, depression, constipation, diarrhea, fluid retention, joint pain, fatigue, thinning hair, menstrual irregularities, rashes, or difficulty losing weight? My guess is more than a few. Did anyone suggest that you may be suffering from food sensitivity, overgrowth of yeast, primarily *Candida*, or parasites? I would guess probably not and if you do have some knowledge of this subject and you have suggested it to your health care provider, it is apt to be quickly dismissed. You know your body better than anyone else. If you suspect that your intestinal barrier is under attack, I would suggest finding a health care practitioner who will take you seriously enough to help you get your life back.

Let's look at food sensitivities a little closer. I am not talking about a food allergy. Those symptoms are very obvious and can be immediately life-threatening for some. Food sensitivities or intolerance have a delayed response that can occur over days. So a symptom you are having today may be related to something you ate three days ago. This makes it very challenging to pin down the offending agent. You can test for some food intolerances in blood, saliva and stool. However, these tests may not show all the foods that you may be having a problem with and this may give you a false sense of security.

These tests are often expensive and not always covered by insurance. However, they can give you a place to start. Checking IgE levels can be a reliable predictor of a food allergy, but not food sensitivity. Using IgG testing will have mixed results and is not always reliable. It is better to look at the leukocyte reactivity in this case as it has been shown to have greater testing sensitivity and validity using this method (Steinman).

The cheapest way to determine if a food is playing havoc with your health is through a food-elimination diet. The top four food intolerances are gluten, milk, eggs, and soy. Ideally you would want to eliminate all four for a period of two months and see if you don't start seeing your symptoms either go away completely or at least significantly improve. However, if you are not willing to do this, than at least start with one of the foods.

You may have developed a food sensitivity to more than one food. This can occur at any point in time in your life and is affected by many of the factors we have discussed throughout this book.

You know what milk, soy, and eggs are, but what is gluten? Gluten is a protein found in wheat, rye, barley, oats, spelt, and kamut. Gluten is used as a filler or sticky substance in many of the processed foods you are buying. It can be hidden in salad dressings, soups, vitamins, makeup, and many other products.

Shockingly ninety-nine percent of those who have gluten sensitivity don't know it. It is a national epidemic related to the high gluten content in genetically-modified grains used in this country. Europe does not allow the use of these grains. We have seen a four-hundred percent increase in the incidence of celiac disease in this country. This is a travesty beyond measure.

Gluten sensitivity may be linked to as many as fifty-five different medical conditions, including heart disease and cancer. This is because gluten is increasing inflammation and inflammation is a known contributor to disease manifestation. If we took just this one problem seriously, think how much health care cost would plummet (Hyman). Not only that, how much healthier we would all be.

It is important to differentiate between gluten sensitivity and celiac disease. Many health care providers and patients alike may confuse them as being the same and they aren't.

A study published in the *American Journal of Gastroenterology, 2011* revealed that gluten sensitivity can be present in the absence of celiac disease. An important distinction between the two is that celiac is a disease and gluten sensitivity causes other diseases to develop. In an ideal world all patients with a chronic health issue of any kind, should be screened for gluten sensitivity (Osborne).

Let me give you an example. I have seen more than one patient come to me that I have felt was a walking poster child for gluten sensitivity. The patient is usually a woman between the ages of thirty-five and fifty-five who has not felt well for a long time. She may have been to several health care providers before ending up on my door step complaining of a host of symptoms, only to be told that she is depressed and needs to lose weight. The typical complaints are foggy thinking, change in mood, extreme fatigue, constipation, joint pain, headaches, menstrual irregularity, sleep disturbance, difficulty losing weight, and swelling hands and feet.

She may have one or more often many of these symptoms. She may be diagnosed with being premenopausal or menopausal, which may also be true but these do not have to result in the symptoms she is having.

She may have developed fibromyalgia, rheumatoid or osteoarthritis, osteoporosis, asthma, high blood pressure, hypothyroidism or a host of other conditions. This may just be the tip of the iceberg, but you get the idea. I might suggest to the patient that she may have an underlying gluten issue and recommend going off gluten for at least a month or two and see if many of her symptoms don't go away. Some take me up on my advice and some don't.

On more than one occasion, when patients take me seriously, they will come back in and say their symptoms are completely gone. How amazing is that? And if they are not completely gone, they are significantly reduced. Now this might not work for everyone, but it is certainly worth a try. I am not going to lie, it is really difficult to follow a gluten-free diet in this highly processed world we live in. However, many who have done this feel so much better. This is motivation enough to keep them away from ever wanting to consume gluten again.

But what if you have tried the gluten-free diet or tried eliminating other foods from your diet and you still are not feeling quite right? The next thing you might want to consider is the possibility that yeast/fungal overgrowth or *Candida albicans* might be playing a role.

The symptoms you can experience with yeast overgrowth are many of the same symptoms you can exhibit with food sensitivities. We all have a certain amount of *Candida* in our digestive tract. When the normal gut flora is thrown out of balance for many of the same reasons previously discussed, this can lead to an overgrowth of yeast.

Many years ago while working as a nurse and before I was a nurse practitioner I asked a physician I was working with at the time if yeast overgrowth could be affecting some of the patients we were seeing. Many had been on antibiotics, steroids, and ate a diet high in refined sugars.

He laughed at me and stated that the only patients that are at risk for an overgrowth of yeast in the form of *Candida albicans* was likely a patient with acquired immune deficiency (AIDS). I didn't argue with him and knew that if I tried to enlighten him on the subject it would have fallen on deaf ears. I also knew that I would never see him as a patient.

The patient walking in my office who I suspect of having yeast overgrowth may have many of the same symptoms as the person with food sensitivities. What may separate them from this group are the presence of dark circles under the eyes, a history of multiple antibiotics or steroids, seasonal allergies, asthma, chronic sinusitis, yeast infections, sleep disturbance, brain fog, anxiety, eczema, and a craving for sugar or carbohydrates. It is very difficult to break the sugar cravings as the little yeasty beasty demands to be fed.

So how do you reduce the yeast overgrowth in your body? It is not easy. First you have to quit feeding it. You do this by cutting out sugars and significantly reducing carbohydrates. In the initial phase this means a very restrictive diet for at least three to four weeks. You don't want to encourage further yeast proliferation. That means no bread, alcohol, or even fruit.

You can have healthy proteins such as eggs, nuts, fish, and lots of non-starchy vegetables. While you are killing off the yeast you want to provide support through foods that promote the repopulation of healthy bacteria. This can be helped by taking a probiotic. You might also want to supplement your diet with natural anti-fungal agents such as garlic, olive leaf extract, oil of oregano, grapefruit seed extract, pau d'acrco tea, caprylic acid, berberine, or extra virgin coconut oil.

Be aware that your symptoms might get worse before they get better as the yeast die-off occurs (Bowden). This is known as herxheimer reaction. As the yeast die off they are releasing toxic substances that trigger an immune response and may intensify the very symptoms you are trying to treat. Indigestion and bloating may initially worsen. It can take up to three-to-four months for the yeast levels to return to normal. In some cases you may need to not only be following a yeast-cleansing diet, but taking prescription antifungal medication and/or supplementation. I also like to use homeopathic agents here as well.

A general three-to-four month protocol to decrease yeast overgrowth would be:

- Eliminate yeast-producing foods and supplements.
- Take a digestive enzyme with every meal. This helps to deter yeast overgrowth in the small intestine.
- Take a probiotic daily on an empty stomach to help repopulate the good bacteria.
- Reduce the burden on the liver as it detoxifies the byproducts from the yeast die-off by taking milk thistle or alpha lipoic acid.

- You may need to be treating an underlying food sensitivity at the same time since the intestinal permeability has been compromised.
- You may need to treat parasites because often where there is yeast, there are parasites.
- Use prescription and natural antifungal agents under the guidance of a trained health care practitioner who is familiar with leaky-gut syndrome or dysbiosis. Some of the natural antifungals are mentioned above. Prescription antifungal may include Diflucan or Nystatin. Prescription antifungal may be needed for six-to-twelve weeks, depending on the situation (Murphree). There are also great homeopathic options available as well.

As I mentioned, where there is yeast there are often parasites. This is the third element I want to discuss that can be invading the mucosal barrier. I can hear you now thinking there *is no way I have parasites!* This only happens to people who have traveled to a foreign country, live in unsanitary conditions, or drink from a poor water supply. I hate to break it to you, but many of us unknowingly are harvesting a healthy population of parasites within our intestinal tract. This can be picked up in the water supply, contaminated foods, and from the soil.

In some cases an undiagnosed parasitic infection can be deadly. Parasites can weaken the immune system and cause fatigue, gastrointestinal pain, body aches and symptoms mimicking chronic fatigue syndrome. It can be difficult to diagnose as the parasites can be very elusive.

Many labs will miss finding parasites in a standard stool test. It is best to have your stool test done at a lab that specializes in parasitology. I have personally seen this in my own practice. When I sent a stool test to the local lab to check for bacteria, ova and parasites the test would be normal. When I sent the test to a lab that specializes in analyzing stool for bacteria, inflammation, and parasites I would get positive lab findings that needed treatment. If your health care provider tells you nothing is wrong and you are still having that chronic diarrhea, constipation, or abdominal pain, get tested by an outside lab. Three good ones that I would recommend are Diagnos-Techs Inc., BioHealth, and Genova Diagnostics. The most common parasites found are giardia, blastocystis hominis, and amebas. If found, these need to be treated with an anti-parasitic agent (Teitelbaum, 133-134).

The third guardian of the digestive tract is the gut-associated lymphoid tissue (GALT). The GALT is not only a very important part of the digestive system, but also of the immune system. It lies underneath the mucosal layer and will seek out and destroy invaders such as bacteria, viruses, and fungi. The GALT also stimulates secretory IgA production which is integral to immune system function (Galland, Lafferty, 25-32).

If this area is compromised through some of the mechanisms we have discussed, this can result in an inflammatory response and breakdown in the ability to fight those invaders.

Then things like food sensitivities and disease develop. This is because the immune system in the gut has been weakened and your secretory IgA has fallen. You can have a reaction to food, the environment, and medications that previously had no ill effects. It is important to remove the irritants that have depleted the level of secretory IgA to the point that now you are having a complete gastrointestinal breakdown. The result of this is disease and weakened immune function. Your quality of life has definitely been affected once you get to this point. The invaders have succeeded in their attack on your natural wall of defenses in the gastrointestinal track. This will result in a domino effect through potentially every system and function in the body.

The repeating theme here is that when any layer of defense within the digestive tract is under attack so too is the immune system. A weakened immune system opens the flood gates of inflammation and disease. There are many ways to help repair and rebuild these natural defenses. To know how to rebuild the digestive tract, it helps to know what caused the breakdown in the first place. This means identifying the root cause. There are many roots to every tree. It can take one or many root causes to bring down that tree and destroy its life source. The same is true for you and me.

There can be one or many causes affecting your health and vitality. To understand what those are may require diagnostic testing to help guide the direction of repairing and rebuilding of not only your digestive tract, but the quality of your life as a whole. You can change your diet, modify stress, work on your emotions and get better quality of sleep and see improvement.

But if there is an underlying parasitic, viral, bacterial, fungal, or hormonal aspect that requires treatment, you don't want to miss it. Specialized testing can help guide the process. This is where supplements and medication may be needed. For example, how are you going to know that you have a low secretory IgA level? You have to be tested. What causes the IgA level to be low? This can be due to adrenal fatigue, hormonal imbalances, food sensitivities, bacterial overgrowth, and a host of other possibilities. To help restore IgA levels, diagnostic testing may be necessary to uncover co-contributing factors. Don't get me wrong; eating a healthy diet and healing underlying emotions and stress are critically important. You will definitely experience significant benefit from addressing these elements. Sometimes though, that is not enough. That is when diagnostic testing can help. It can also help direct the approach you take on your path to health and healing.

One thing that we have not yet talked about when addressing gastrointestinal health is detoxification. Detoxification is the body's way of removing toxins from within and outside the body. This is a complex process that requires an orchestra of players including not only the gastrointestinal tract, but also the help from other parts of the digestive, respiratory, circulatory, lymphatic, integumentary (skin), and urinary systems as well. Put another way is that the liver, lungs, heart, blood vessels, drainage pipes (lymph), skin, and kidneys all have to play nice together. The detoxification pathway can be blocked by genetics, poor diet, stress, medications, illness, and all of the other things previously discussed. I don't mean to sound like a broken record, but the body is like an orchestra. If one instrument is out of tune, everything else in the production is off.

Many of the things we have talked about up to this point can help to improve how well the body naturally clears toxins. However, sometimes the line of communication breaks down and in spite of your best efforts, there is a glitch in the detoxification pathway. We are all genetically different and therefore metabolize things very differently as well. You and I can be exposed to the same things, but can have very different reactions to how the body clears the toxic elements from our bodies. I might be a fast metabolizer and you may be a slow metabolizer.

For example, let's say we both are exposed to mold. As a fast metabolizer my body, after inhaling the toxic mold, is able to detoxify it out very quickly with little to no ill effects. You as the slow metabolizer have an inflammatory response and it takes you a week to recover from the brief exposure to mold. It is the difference between pouring water through a funnel versus a skinny straw. It is just going to take longer to get the same amount of water through the straw as it is the funnel.

Many of your Eastern medicines, such as Traditional Chinese Medicine, promote a diet that supports natural detoxification and often recommends cleansing or fasting. When considering a more comprehensive detoxification that goes beyond some of the lifestyle factors we have discussed, I would recommend working with a trained practitioner. There can be many layers to this process and lots of toxic garbage to be cleared out after years of exposure. It is like peeling away the layers of an onion, one layer at a time until you reach the core. You can't get to the core without clearing away the other layers.

Before I consider putting someone on a comprehensive detoxification program I will do a thorough assessment. I am going to want to know what medications you are taking. What illnesses you have or have had. What kind of diet you are eating. Do you smoke or drink? What is your family history? Have you had any surgery? What environmental risk factors you might have. I will likely want to obtain some baseline laboratory information. There are many things to consider as I want to put the body in the best possible state to get the most out of the detoxification process. That is not to say people don't do this without help, but sometimes, if this process is not done right in someone who is vulnerable, it may create more problems for that person.

Before putting someone on a detoxification program, I will have done a physical examination and diagnostic testing to look for root factors or underlying causes. I am back to that root system again. Then, before beginning any deep cleansing program you may be asked to make certain dietary and environmental changes and asked to work on underlying stress and emotional blocks. This just helps to decrease some of the inflammation within the detoxification pathways. If you try to detox before improving the foundation, how well do you think things are going to hold up over the long haul? Probably not well.

Sure, you may either feel sicker or revitalize, but those losses or gains are going to be short-lived. This initial detoxification phase will likely take three months. During this time you will be working to repair and repopulate the gut. It is in the second phase of detoxification that a deep cleanse is recommended to open the system up further. This is where I would recommend a supplemental regimen to aid in the process now that you have reinforced the foundation. You will get so much more out of this process by doing this and are going to feel so much better. You will likely feel better than you have in years. Now when talking about detoxification here, I am not talking about colonics. For me, a slow and gentle approach is better for long-term gains.

There is no fasting involved. You will be advised to follow a healthy diet and supplemental support may also be recommended at this phase as well. This phase also takes around three months to complete. In the third phase you want to go even deeper to address things like yeast and parasites if necessary. Every situation is different and the pace and program is very individualized. For most, detoxification can take three-to-six months of slow steady work. There are all kinds of ways to detoxify. Some are better than others. I am sharing with you what I have found to work well for long term gains, not short term reward. Ultimately it is up to you to decide how and when to clean out your own closet.

So what are some ways to help promote limiting your toxic burden and optimizing your detoxification pathways now and in the future? Limit your dietary and environmental exposure. Eat a healthy diet by eliminating processed foods, artificial sweeteners and excessive alcohol and caffeine. Use natural cleaning products. Don't smoke. Avoid exposure to pesticides, mold, and radiation. Limit exposure to electromagnetic fields. Exercise is a natural detoxifier and promotes lymphatic drainage. Drink plenty of filtered water. Breathe deeply and consider using an infrared sauna to expel and sweat out the toxins. Adequate fiber can help promote daily bowel movements. Eliminate unnecessary medications through the guidance of your health care practitioner. Consider detoxifying juicing with various vegetables and fruits.

There are certain foods that help promote detoxification such as avocados, berries, artichokes, beets, leafy greens, dandelion, broccoli, cauliflower, cabbage, garlic, oregano, parsley, and others (Mullin, Swift, 124). Fresh is best. Eat close to the earth and eat organic.

Take Away Tips: GI and Detox
- A healthy gut equals and healthy body and mind.
- Repopulate the gut with healthy bacteria-promoting foods and probiotics.

- Heal the mucosal lining by eliminating inflammatory agents.
- Look for the root cause through diagnostic testing.
- Identify and eliminate food sensitivities.
- Complete a comprehensive detoxification program.

Hormones

Have you ever been told it's just your hormones? Does this infuriate you? It very well can be your hormones that are out of control and making you feel tired, moody, irritable, impacting your sleep, making it difficult for you to lose weight, causing breast tenderness, lowering your libido or sex drive, and affecting your menstrual cycle or contributing to erectile dysfunction.

Is this really what we have to look forward to as we age? This can be your fate only if you allow it to be. Life is all about choices. You can accept the idea that this is a normal part of aging, or you can choose to reject this notion and do something about it. It is really up to you. We have a choice to speed up the aging process by not living a fulfilled life of purpose and burying our emotions in poor lifestyle habits, or we can live consciously and nurture the seed of life in ourselves to live a healthy, long and vital life. We greatly increase our odds by actively applying many of the principles highlighted throughout this book. I bring this up here because if we don't apply them as we age, the hormonal breakdown that seems to hit most in midlife will occur. To what degree varies from person to person.

I have seen many women and men hit the middle of life feeling worn out. They have no energy, sex becomes a chore, their memory is not what it used to be, they are struggling to lose weight, hair is falling out in one place and growing in places you don't want it to grow, they are tired but can't sleep. Does any of this sound familiar? This is what happens when the cumulative effects of years of stress, poor diet, emotional baggage, and environmental exposures lead to hormonal burnout and collapse.

All the hormones in the body comprise what is known as the endocrine system. Each endocrine gland performs a function and produces hormones. One hormone will affect the action of another hormone. Hormones function interdependently, not independently. Hormones are stimulated into action by everything we have been talking about including age, gender, genetics, environment, stress, diet, food sensitivities, and emotions. The endocrine system function is also interconnected to the immune and nervous systems. So as you can see, there are many things that can determine how hormonally balanced we are.

The endocrine system has many working parts that are in constant communication. The endocrine glands are the pineal, hypothalamus, pituitary, parathyroid, thyroid, thymus, stomach, adrenal, pancreas, ovaries, and testes. Within the endocrine system releasing hormones trigger stimulating hormones to tell a target gland to produce a hormone to respond and create an action that will then tell another hormone to do the same process. The hypothalamus-pituitary-adrenal axis (HPA axis) is the primary feedback loop responsible.

There are branches that feed off of this main feedback loop and when there is a system breakdown or hormone imbalance, there has been a block that has occurred causing this system to derail somewhere along its natural path.

We also need cholesterol in healthy amounts, believe it or not, to make this system work. All hormones are derived from cholesterol. You read that right. All hormones are derived from cholesterol. The diagram below from *Functional Diagnostic Nutrition* shows the complexity of this system. What I want you to understand by looking at this diagram is one hormone breaks down to another hormone and each hormone has a function.

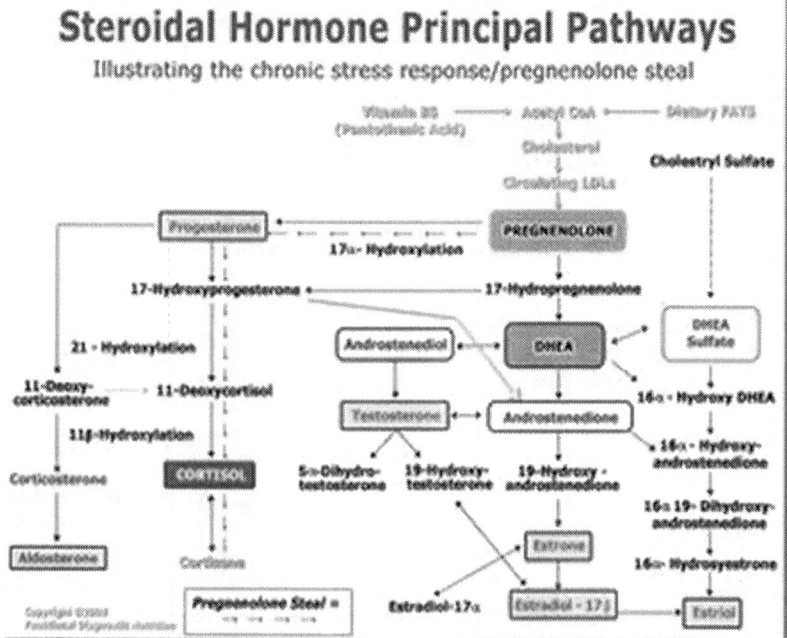

There are five main classes of hormone groups: glucocorticoids, mineralcorticoids, androgens, estrogens, and progestagens. Glucocorticoids are important in controlling inflammation and immune function. They also can affect metabolism and cortisol release from the adrenal glands. Mineralcorticoids have a direct impact on water and electrolyte balance. Androgen hormones are dehyydroepiandrosterone (DHEA) and testosterone and can affect aging, memory, vitality, bone density, and libido. Progesterone is the primary progestagen and is vitally important to menstrual cycles and sustaining a pregnancy. It has many functions that we will elaborate on further. Estrogens also affect menstrual cycles and pregnancy, but also bone density and memory. I will expand upon this as well (McEvoy).

There are many other hormone groups such as insulin, human growth hormone, and thyroid hormones. Whole books are dedicated to discussing the complexity and science of hormone function. I just want to help you understand the function of a few key hormones. To remind you, emotional blocks, stress and poor diet are at the root of all health issues, including hormonal balance.

The powerhouse gland is the adrenal. If the adrenal glands are not functioning optimally, we are going to be on a downward slope trying to hold onto our health. We have two small adrenal glands sitting atop each kidney that are truly miraculous little organs. The adrenals help maintain balance and harmony within, control sleep-wake cycles, energy level, weight and metabolism, emotions, stress response, and impact almost all body functions.

Several key hormones are produced by the adrenal glands. From cholesterol, as noted in the diagram previously, we get pregnenolone. Pregnenolone is the building block of progesterone, and DHEA which convert to cortisol, estrogen, and testosterone. Pregnenolone is vital to brain function and nerve regeneration. Stress will have an effect on its production. If pregnenolone production is decreased, all the other hormones just listed will decrease as well.

To break this down further we will look at each hormone individually along with its function.

Progesterone is one of the two main hormones associated with female reproduction and the menstrual cycle. It is produced by the ovaries and to a lesser degree the adrenals and even the testes in men. It effects and is affected by other hormones including estrogen, cortisol, testosterone, and aldosterone. No pregnancy can be sustained without adequate progesterone as it is vital to the health of the endometrium (uterine lining) inside and outside of pregnancy.

Progesterone has many benefits outside of the sex organs including acting as a mild diuretic, fat metabolism, mood, thyroid function, blood clotting, blood sugar regulation, cell oxygenation, skin moisture, zinc and copper levels, and libido. It also provides protection against breast cysts, breast cancer, uterine cancer, and decreases estrogen dominance. When we go through menopause, it is assumed that the unpleasant symptoms are solely due to low estrogen.

Progesterone levels actually fall before estrogen levels creating an imbalance between the two. That is why many women in the premenopause period feel hormonally out of balance. It is why so many women also experience what is known as estrogen dominance. In men, progesterone is a precursor of testosterone and corticosteroids and remains somewhat constant well into their seventies and eighties.

Progesterone is converted to cortisol a glucocorticoid that is vitally important to sustaining life. Cortisol levels are integral to a normal circadian rhythm or sleep-wake cycle. Cortisol levels should be higher in the morning and steadily decline by the evening hours. Unfortunately in many the normal circadian rhythm will get out of balance. You can end up having high cortisol levels at night and this can lead to insomnia or difficulty sleeping. You may have low cortisol levels in the morning when they should be highest and struggle to get out of bed and get to work on time.

Stress and emotions are intimately related to cortisol levels and overall health as we learned when we talked about stress earlier. If there is a time of day when you are fatigued or anxious this may be a sign of cortisol imbalance that is affecting your emotional and physical health. For example, in applying the Five Element Theory, let's say you wake up every night at two a.m. and you always have trouble getting back to sleep. This can be a sign of unresolved anger or frustration. It may also be a sign of liver issues, such as fatty liver disease which is epidemic in the country. This is due to poor diet and stress.

Closely tied to cortisol and the stress response are aldosterone, epinephrine and norepinephrine which are also produced by the adrenal glands. Aldosterone is important to maintaining fluid balance, sodium, potassium, and blood pressure regulation. The adrenaline produced from epinephrine and norepinephrine regulates blood pressure, heart rate, blood vessel and airway constriction or dilation, muscle tension or relaxation, mood, and metabolism.

Excessive stimulation and chronic elevation of cortisol and adrenaline will suppress immune function, slow down metabolism and increase weight, increase blood pressure and raise the risks of heart disease. Over stimulation of cortisol and adrenaline causes the liver to produce more glucose (blood sugar) and the pancreas to work harder to crank out more insulin leading to insulin resistance and diabetes (Simpson, 5-48).

There will be a deterioration of the HPA axis communication system with misfires or messages that are not received. Thyroid hormone production is a common casualty as the adrenal glands begin to burnout.

Adrenal fatigue is a common term used to describe what happens when the adrenal glands just can't keep up. Cortisol and adrenaline levels start to fall and cause overwhelming fatigue and in some a low or high blood pressure, weight loss or gain, emotional chaos, and low or high blood sugar levels. Cortisol is necessary for energy production, metabolism, blood sugar regulation, mood, immune function, and the rate at which we age. Healthy cortisol levels are vital to disease prevention.

Adrenal health is closely tied to thyroid health. The thyroid gland is equally as important as the adrenal gland as it affects the regulation of other hormones and body systems function. If your thyroid hormone begins to produce too little or too much thyroid hormone you can feel miserable. A low functioning thyroid (hypothyroidism) will slow everything down. You may feel fatigue (tired), have foggy thinking, constipation, joint pain, weight gain, elevated cholesterol, dry skin, menstrual irregularities, fluid retention, hair loss, depression, cold intolerance, decreased sweating, brittle nails, headaches, decreased libido, heart palpitations, difficulty swallowing, infertility, low body temperature, fluid retention, muscle weakness, and blood pressure changes (R. Shames, Shames, 51-58).

A thyroid that is producing too much thyroid hormone is known as hyperthyroidism. With hyperthyroidism everything is sped up. This can result in excessive sweating, diarrhea, elevated blood pressure, heart palpitations, insomnia, irritability and mood swings, tremors, weight loss, fatigue, feeling hot, increased appetite, and muscle weakness. This is most commonly seen with what is known as Graves's disease.

The next hormone we are going to talk about is DHEA. DHEA results from the conversion of pregnenolone and is the most abundant hormone. DHEA is important to brain function, energy level, immune function, and affects aging and inflammation. DHEA levels are highest as we are growing and begin to decline as early as the late twenties. By the time we are in our seventies we may have only five-to-ten percent of the DHEA we had in our twenties.

In order to try and hold on to their youth many people will purchase over the counter DHEA. I would caution you against this even though I know many natural practitioners often recommend or prescribe DHEA to their clients. Too much DHEA can cause hair to grow where you might not want it, greasy skin and hair, excess body odor, aggression, mood swings, acne, and a deepening voice.

It can also potentially convert to the protective estrogen known as estriol, or it could convert to an excess of estrone, and estradiol thereby increasing your risks of uterine or breast cancer. Supplementation may also cause a decrease in the natural production of DHEA, making the body too reliant on the need for supplementation. My advice would be to not supplement with DHEA, but if you do, work with a practitioner who can measure and monitor your steroidal hormone pathways.

DHEA levels can be directly affected by gut inflammation, secretory IgA and cortisol levels. Secretory IgA and cortisol are affected by stress and diet.

From DHEA estrogen and testosterone are produced. Estrogens are produced in the adrenals and the ovaries primarily.

There are three main types of estrogen, estrone, estradiol, and estriol. Estriol is the weakest of the estrogens and has protective qualities against breast and uterine cancer. Estrone and estradiol are the more potent of the estrogens and are involved in the development of secondary sex characteristics such as breast development. Estrogen is very interrelated with progesterone in regulating the menstrual cycle.

Estrogen, like adrenal function, can interfere with thyroid hormones, body fat, sex drive, fluid retention, blood sugar control, cardiovascular tone, autoimmune disorders, bone density, blood clotting, and impact breast and uterine cancer development. As you may recall, when a woman approaches menopause her progesterone levels nose dive before the estrogen levels begin to fall. This can set the stage for estrogen dominance. Estrogen dominance generally will affect women between the ages of thirty-five to fifty. However with the growing obesity epidemic in this country, women can have estrogen dominance issues much earlier because fat cells love to hold on to estrogen. It is the unpleasant side effects of estrogen dominance that will often cause women to seek out help from their health care practitioner as they are desperate to feel normal.

Many of the symptoms of estrogen dominance are very much like the symptoms you can see with hypothyroidism. Do you feel like you aged overnight? This is often a time when you may also develop food or environmental allergies that you did not previously have. I have even seen women develop asthma.

Other symptoms associated with estrogen dominance may be breast tenderness, fibrocystic breasts, decreased libido, depression, fatigue, foggy thinking, headaches, increased blood clotting, infertility, irritability, memory loss, miscarriage, osteoporosis, premenstrual symptoms, uterine fibroids, increased fat distribution and weight gain around the abdomen, gall bladder disease, breast or uterine cancer, and autoimmune disease (Lee, Hopkins, 34-43).

Testosterone is derived from DHEA and progesterone. This is the main sex hormone in men, but it is also produced in women to a lesser degree. Men go through their own form of menopause or andropause beginning in their forties as their testosterone levels begin to decline. Men with low testosterone can have decrease muscle mass, depression, fatigue, decrease libido, erectile dysfunction, memory loss, weight gain, and have an increased incidence of diabetes, and cardiovascular disease.

In women testosterone can also affect libido and even cardiovascular function, bone density, memory, and immune function. Too much testosterone can affect immune function, prostate cancer in men, and lead to obesity, polycystic ovaries, facial hair and acne in women (Braverman, 220-231).

If you suspect that you are having a hormonal issue, how do you fix it? First and foremost you have to work on managing stress and changing your diet. If these two key areas are not addressed, taking a supplement or using synthetic or natural hormones are not going to effectively help to regain control and balance to your hormonal health. That is not to say that certain supplements and preferably natural hormone therapy cannot aid in this process, but you have to address the underlying cause.

The underlying cause is often related to a combination of all of the things we have been talking about, including stress, diet, gastrointestinal health, emotions, adequate sleep, food sensitivities, and environment.

Ideally, I would recommend you work with a trained holistic practitioner to help identify some of the root causes and the specific imbalances you may have. Your practitioner can assess your situation, recommend appropriate diagnostic testing, and help you formulate a treatment plan to support your path to health and healing.

We learned from the Women's Health Initiative (WHI) study that hormone replacement therapy (HRT) is nothing to mess with and can be detrimental to one's health. In the WHI study it was determined that women who were on HRT in the form of combination synthetic estrogen and progestin were at an increased risk of breast cancer, ovarian cancer, heart disease, blood clots in the lungs, stroke, and gall bladder disease (Schneider, Hirschman, 128-130).

There is still a debate going on regarding the results of this study several years later. I will share some supplements that can provide support to your hormone balance. There are supplements geared to treat a particular symptom such as hot flashes. I do think if you address the underlying root cause, things like hot flashes, sleep disturbances, weight gain and mood swings will improve on their own. That is why working with a trained practitioner to help determine your hormone levels is so important.

I prefer saliva testing. I feel this test is more sensitive to revealing the correlation between your actual symptoms and hormone picture. Saliva testing will reveal what your unbound active hormone levels are and in my experience this has correlated well with the patient's actual symptoms. There are many potential treatment options to relieve the unpleasant affects of hormone imbalance. I will be giving you a few, well researched options that promote balance versus a specific symptom relief, such as hot flashes. Keep in mind that a supplement is not a replacement for a healthy diet, exercise, adequate sleep, addressing your emotional blocks, or stress management.

Estrogen dominance is a common problem that many women face. This is created when estrogen is out of balance with progesterone. To help encourage a healthy estrogen balance and get rid of excess harmful estrogens there are some supplements that can help to support this effort. One of the best ways to do this is by eating a lot of cruciferous vegetables such as broccoli, cauliflower, brussel sprouts, and cabbage. These cruciferous vegetables contain a substance known as indole-3-carbinole that helps detoxify excess and potentially carcinogenic forms of estrogen.

You can buy indole-3-carbinole in a supplement, but it is unstable in this form. If you are going to take a supplement that augments the benefits of indole-3-carbinole, you should take diindolymethane (DIM). DIM helps to decrease the bad 16-hydroxyestrone and increase the good 2-hydroxyestrone. As a result DIM can help alleviate breast tenderness, menstrual pain, and premenstrual symptoms. A dose of 30mg daily is like eating two pounds of broccoli.

Calcium D-glucarate also helps promote healthy estrogen metabolism by eliminating excess estradiol. It also promotes healthy cell development and inhibits glucoronidase release. Glucoronidase slows down the detoxification of harmful cancer-causing substances. A dose of 200mg once or twice daily may be suggested.

To support progesterone levels, consider chaste berry, also known as Vitex. Chaste berry is believed to stimulate the pituitary to release more luteinizing hormone which then stimulates progesterone production. A dose of 20 to 25 mg daily is recommended (Lucille, 23-25). Progesterone cream is widely available over the counter. However, I don't recommend using it because you could make an already existing hormone imbalance worse.

We are trying to restore balance. That is not to say there aren't those of you out there that have tried over the counter progesterone cream and report feeling better. However, remember we are trying to address the root cause or causes. Rubbing progesterone cream on your body without knowing if that is what your body needs may in fact be covering up what needs to be uncovered.

A temporary fix does not result in a long-term solution. I have seen many women come into my practice who report having felt great initially, but eventually they ended up using more and more of the cream to try to hold on to the initial effect. Next thing you know they are in a bigger hormonal mess than where they started. You want to encourage long-term balance, not chronic imbalance.

I do feel homeopathy is a great source to help restore hormone balance. Homeopathy has been around for hundreds of years and is the second most used medical system in the world. I have seen many women and even some men regain hormonal balance with homeopathic support. Homeopathy, as you may recall, was discussed when talking about supplements. However it is worth reviewing here.

Homeopathy is from two Greek words, homoios: meaning similar and pathos: meaning suffering. The word homeopathy was first coined by Samuel Hahnemann, the founder of modern homeopathy. Homeopathy means like cures like or what created the imbalance can also cure the imbalance. Homeopathic medicines are micro-dosed natural substances derived from botanical, animal or mineral sources. The medicine is diluted or de-concentrated and then vigorously shaken, traditionally referred to as succussion. This process transforms the original substance into a therapeutically-active medicine.

Homeopathy is a safe and natural method to balance the body and allow the body to heal. Incredibly small amounts of homeopathic substances are needed to aid in healing. They are so diluted down that many argue they have no actual active ingredient. It is the reported energy of the substance that helps to restore balance.

I know this may be a stretch for some of you to wrap your head around. I understand and appreciate that. It would not have sustained the test of time if there was not something to its powerful effect. Homeopathies can indeed be quite powerful and an amazing means to restoring balance and healing.

To help you in selecting a homeopathy there are some basic things you want to know. Keep in mind though that homeopathy is not a simple science and people study for years to perfect the art and science of homeopathy. Having said that, if you are buying one of the widely available over-the-counter remedies, there are some basics you want to know when selecting a remedy and strength. So let's review again what those are.

Simillimum refers to identifying a remedy that most closely matches to a person's set of unique symptoms. Potency is the strength of a homeopathic remedy. For example, you will see the potencies referred to as, 12X, 6C, 30C, 10M or 6LM. X potencies stay in the body a short period of time and can be used safely for repeat dosing. X potencies are used for 1st aid, trauma, recovery from injury, preventative dosing, sudden illness, seasonal problems, and general family use. C potencies are used for first aid, seasonal ailments and chronic health concerns. M potency is used for health problems or constitutional treatment.

Very high potencies may stay working in the body for months. High LM potencies are very popular and safe for dealing with children's ailments, sensitive people and emotional issues (Dale). There are numerous scientific studies that have been done using homeopathic agents. In fact, several studies have confirmed that homeopathies are biologically active. I have safely used homeopathy to restore hormonal balance in women that have had breast cancer.

To give you an example, a woman came into the practitioner with a history of breast cancer. She had been on bio-identical hormone therapy. This was after being diagnosed and treated for her breast cancer. This is something I would not recommend. She was suffering with several menopausal symptoms. When her hormone levels were checked, she was found to have dangerously elevated levels of the most potent estrogens of estrone and estradiol.

This excess estrogen no doubt was a contributing factor to her breast cancer. I do not know of one single physician who ever checks the hormone levels of the women he is treating for breast cancer. If they did and encouraged hormone balancing options, it begs the question if we wouldn't see more breast cancer survivor success stories.

Now getting back to our lady with the history of breast cancer, through a comprehensive review of her entire hormone picture, an individualized treatment plan for her included the use of homeopathy, among other things, to bring down the level of excess estrogen. On a retest after months of treatment, her estrone and estradiol levels were restored and brought back into a normal safe range. The menopausal symptoms she was having - hot flashes, sleep disturbance, and fatigue - resolved or were significantly improved. I have seen this kind of response to homeopathic treatments many times in my own practice and that is why I am a fan of homeopathy. I have seen women regain hormone balance, and their unpleasant menopausal symptoms such as hot flashes, irritability, and poor sleep alleviated.

Testosterone support can be achieved with homeopathy as well. DHEA is a popular supplement used to support testosterone levels. As I mentioned earlier, I don't generally recommend this but do in rare instances but only after evaluating an individual's hormonal pathways. You can do more harm than good here if you aren't careful. One potential supporting element to testosterone imbalance that you may not have heard of is *Eurycoma longifolia*. I would consider using that before I would DHEA. Eurycoma is believed to assist in bringing suboptimal testosterone levels back into balance.

It does this not by increasing testosterone production, but by freeing up testosterone from sex hormone-binding globulin. The result is improved mood, energy, mental focus, and libido. Recommended dose is 50-100mg per day of water-extracted eurycoma root. *Cordyceps sinensis* is a Chinese mushroom that has been used for centuries to treat fatigue and improve lung function. More recent studies have shown that it can also help restore testosterone levels to normal. A dose of two-to-four grams daily is considered safe.

Another key component to restoring hormonal balance, if not the most important, is adrenal support. I don't believe you can fully restore estrogen and progesterone balance without adrenal support. Remember the HPA axis. If there is a break in communication in that feedback loop, you are going to continue to have problems. Supplements that have been shown to support adrenal function are commonly referred to as adaptogens. Several ginseng varieties have been shown to support adrenal function. These include *Indian ginseng* (ashwaganda), *Chinese ginseng* (Panax ginseng), and *Siberian ginseng* (Eleuthercoccus senticosus).

Ginseng helps to restore cortisol balance, and boost energy. Dosage will depend on the type of ginseng used and specific needs of the individual. *Rhodiola rosea* is another adaptogen that is believed to aid the body in its response to psychological and physiological stress. It is considered to be safe and helpful in restoring energy and decreasing fatigue without being a stimulant. General dosage recommendations are 300-600mg daily (Talbott, 218-227).

There are several key nutrients that help support adrenal function and enhance the effect of any adaptogen you may use, in particular vitamins B and C. So consuming a diet that is rich in healthy vitamins and minerals is going to further support healthy adrenal gland function.

In order to support thyroid function you have to have healthy adrenals. You may have heard that iodine, L-tyrosine, selenium, and zinc are important to thyroid function. So what do you do, you run out and buy one or all of these and start taking them hoping it will help improve your already poorly-functioning thyroid. But unless you are supporting your adrenal glands, that thyroid is going to have to continue to work extra hard. Having said that, why are these substances important to thyroid function?

Iodine in combination with L-tyrosine is necessary for thyroid hormone production and the conversion of T4 to the active thyroid hormone, T3. Thyroid hormone metabolism is also supported by selenium. Selenium is a very important trace mineral that helps to create a very powerful antioxidant known as glutathione that helps as a scavenger for free radicals involved in inflammation and disease. A healthy glutathione pathway supports body detoxification (Lucille, 66-67). When this pathway is working well, thyroid hormone production improves. These nutrients ideally should not be taken in excessively high amounts. If you have Hashimoto's thyroiditis and are taking mega doses of any one of these substances, you may actually decrease instead of enhance your thyroid function.

The subject of mega doses of iodine has been debated within and outside of the natural health care arena. I would be cautious and if at all possible, get your nutrient levels tested before taking high doses. Again this is where getting your iodine, L-tyrosine, and selenium from food sources and a comprehensive multivitamin is your safest bet.

As you can see your hormonal production and its associated pathways are very complex. There are so many variables involved and one little detour in that pathway can throw you completely off track. There is more to your hormones than your age or whether you are pre or post menopausal. The three undiscovered pathways we started off this chapter with stress, gastrointestinal health, and detoxification are intimately connected to hormonal balance. So taking a pill to increase your libido, or rubbing on a cream to alleviate hot flashes often is not going to be very successful if you aren't addressing those other factors as well.

Take Away Tips

- Hormones make up what is known as the endocrine system. Hormones work together to maintain balance.
- Progesterone helps regulate the menstrual cycle, maintain a pregnancy, regulate metabolism, is protective against breast and uterine cancer, and has an affect mood, sleep and libido. Chaste berry is believed to stimulate progesterone production at a dose of 20-to 25-mg daily.

- Estrogen, like progesterone, helps to regulate the menstrual cycle, can affect thyroid function, body fat, sex drive, fluid retention, blood sugar control, cardiovascular tone, autoimmune disorders, bone density, blood clotting, and impact breast and uterine cancer development. Symptoms of estrogen dominance are your warning sign that your hormones are out of balance. Cruciferous vegetables or DIM in a dose of 30mg daily can help reduce or prevent estrogen excess.

- Testosterone is the primary sex hormone in men and has an effect on muscle mass, mood, energy, libido, memory, weight, blood sugar regulation, and cardiovascular health. In women testosterone can also affect libido and even cardiovascular function, bone density, memory, and immune function. Eurycoma 50-100mg daily or Cordyceps two-to-four grams daily may help to regulate testosterone levels.

- Cortisol levels are integral to a normal circadian rhythm or sleep-wake cycle and are an important measure of adrenal health. To restore hormonal balance, the adrenal glands always need support.

Ginseng or Rhodiola are both known as adaptogens and support adrenal function balance.

- DHEA is important to brain function, energy level, immune function, and affects aging and inflammation. I don't recommend supplemental DHEA but on rare occasion.
- Thyroid function is dependent on adrenal function. A diet rich in iodine, selenium, and L-tyrosine helps support thyroid function.
- Homeopathy is a safe option to help in restoring hormonal balance.

CHAPTER EIGHT
Change

Up to now all you have been reading about is change. How do I change my life so that I feel better, have more energy, and live longer? You might be thinking change is hard. You are right, change is hard. However, if change does not occur you are going to continue to feel like you do right now. If you remain in the same stagnant patterns, it is like stepping into quicksand.

Putting things off until tomorrow, next week or next year will only keep you stuck. Your health and well-being are the same. Only you can make the choice to stay stuck until your health sinks beyond the point of no return or you can throw out the lifeline and rescue yourself.

Fight for your health and stop making excuses as to why you are stuck or blaming others for your situation. This will only leaves you stuck. Don't keep giving your power to succeed away by finding excuses as to why you can't achieve optimal health and healing. Set aside the excuses and instead ask how do I begin to make a beneficial change?

Will it be scary? Absolutely! Is it necessary? Yes, if you want to free yourself from the limitations you have placed on yourself. I hope you give serious thought to making permanent lifestyle changes. Not for me. Not for your family or friends. For any change to be successful, it needs to come from within you for you.

Only you can change you!

No one gets through life without having to make adjustments to adapt to things that change our lives. Avoidance is a fear-based emotion that can keep you from fully experiencing life. Fear literally means, " *Frozen Ego Awaiting Release*."

How many times have you avoided doing something because you were afraid? Often this ego-based fear can be fear of failure, fear of not being liked, fear of success, fear of being hurt, or fear of feeling your emotions. There are probably thousands of fears one could come up with. Fear is an emotion that must be faced head-on in order for personal transformation to occur. Move out of your fear and embrace change. Change is an opportunity to learn and grow. We are always evolving.

It is our lack of self-confidence or self-worth that keeps us locked in our own fear. This will leave you paralyzed and keep you from moving forward and down the yellow brick road to self-transformation. Fear is an emotionally-based thought of self-victimization. In order to let this go requires self love and acceptance, faults and all. Find your inner courage, just like the cowardly lion did in the *Wizard of Oz*. Move out of your head, the ego, and into the heart of who you were always meant to be.

In order to start making changes in your health it all may seem overwhelming at this point. Many studies and books have been written on change and what change means. Certainly we could explore various ideas on change and how to go about making a change in our personal lives or business.

Let's look at one example of the steps involved in making a change by James Prochaska, a well-known health-promotion change theorist. Prochaska's theory can be applied to all aspects of life in regards to health improvement. This is whether you are trying to make a lifestyle change or defining something as deep as your life's purpose.

According to Prochaska's Theoretical Model for Change, there are six stages of change one goes through. The six stages of change include pre-contemplation, contemplation, preparation, action, maintenance, and termination. Now you don't have to be versed in stuffy theories or memorize the steps given here. You are likely already consciously or subconsciously applying the different steps of change through your own thoughts and planning.

But if you are going to seriously start taking steps forward it does help to have a plan of action. Even if you don't have a formal plan of action, just making a conscious commitment to make a change may be good enough.

So how do we apply Prochaska's stages of change to a path to health and healing? How do we plant the seeds for change within ourselves? Let's look at each stage of change and how it applies to making a bad habit or habits that are no longer serving us into a good habits or life changing experiences.

There are different ideas of how long this process can take and they will be dependent on the habit you are trying to change. Each of us is unique and while it may take one person only a couple of weeks to change a personal goal, it can take another person three months or three years to achieve.

In other cases it may take a lifetime. It is dependent on what it is you are trying to change and your motivation for personal transformation. You may have setbacks and move back and forth between various stages. Don't give up. Don't beat yourself up. Just keep trying. The only failure is in not having tried at all. It can take one try or it may take one-hundred tries to reach your goal. Find your path and if you get detoured, find your way back as soon as possible. A path, as in life, can have many hills, valleys, twists, and turns. Forge ahead and just keep moving. Einstein once said that, "We are boxed in by the boundary conditions of our thinking". If you think you can't make a change you won't, and you will continue to get what you have always gotten. Change your way of thinking and looking at yourself and the world around you. You may then journey down a path you never dreamed possible.

So what is the definition Prochaska gave to each stage of change and how do I apply that to my own path to health and healing?

During the pre-contemplation stage you are not even thinking about making a lifestyle change. You may be in denial or unaware of a real or potential health issue. It is possible at this stage that you are becoming aware that there is a problem and that certain aspects of your life are out of control. You are in survival mode with no clear plan or direction. At this stage you may also be able to give multiple excuses why now is not a good time to make a change. You can procrastinate yourself literally to death.

For example, let's say you have put on twenty pounds in the last year and have moved into elastic waist pants. Your habits don't otherwise change and it has not occurred to you maybe even that you have put on twenty pounds or you have chosen to ignore it. You happen to get weighed at your company's health screening and you might be thinking you have gained a couple of pounds since the last health screening. When you are told you have gained twenty pounds you are shocked and can't believe it. The scale must be wrong. There is no way that is correct. You demand to be weighed on a different scale.

You are advised to consider losing weight. How insulting? That scale is wrong. No change is made at this point. Six months later you are seeing your health care provider and asked to get on the scale so a weight can be obtained. You are told you are now twenty-five pounds heavier than you were only a year and a half ago. Your health care provider walks into the room and voices concern about the change in your weight. What has happened in the past year? Are you going through menopause? Are you not sleeping well? What emotional baggage are you carrying around? What cravings are you feeding? What stressful events have taken place?

At this point you are advised of the health risks and are also told your blood pressure has gone up. You are now faced with the reality that the scale during the health screen you had six months ago was right after all. Your consciousness has now been raised. You either see this as a wakeup call or you get mad at your health care provider because you feel embarrassed and insulted.

You can stay stuck in your path at this point or start contemplating making a change and choosing a different path. Thought patterns that will leave you stuck and unable to move forward include: denial, blame, self-criticism, resentment, fear, or a host of other emotions. Identify the emotional pattern that is preventing you from moving forward. Get out of your own way. Step out of your ego. Yes, this can leave you feeling vulnerable. It also can be extremely liberating as you break through the wall that is holding you back from expressing your true self. To shed the pounds or change a habit successfully will require unleashing the emotional blocks that are keeping you stuck.

I hope you have chosen to face your fears and forge ahead. Once your consciousness has been raised and the reality of the situation has set in, you have entered the contemplation stage and really start thinking about the weight you have gained. You also begin to formulate an idea about how you are going to lose the weight or you could be coming up with excuses why you can't lose the weight.

There's that emotional block again. What are the pros and cons of different methods to getting the weight off? How do you make a change that can lead to permanent weight loss? You might surf the Internet looking for the latest weight loss pill or diet program. You may read one or several books on the latest fat-burning craze. Perhaps you are considering joining one of the local weight loss groups.

Ideally you will be doing some self analysis. What got you to this place? What emotion are you trying to feed or heal? In order to make long-lasting changes to achieving your goal your emotional health must be addressed. This is a time of inner reflection and a time to make a serious reality check. It is also important to ask yourself why. Why do you want to make this change now? Asking why forces you to look at the emotional attachments that have prevented you from taking action or sticking with a program in the past.

The contemplation stage is the information-gathering and thinking stage. You may even be thinking about formulating a plan or goal to set about losing the weight.

In stage three, preparation, you are now ready to move forward and may tell friends and family you are changing your eating and exercise habits. This is the time to develop a plan of action. Be ready to roll up your sleeves and dive in.

You might start looking for or have identified a diet support group or fitness center to join. Maybe you buy a cookbook geared towards healthy eating. You have set a date to begin your journey. A year has now past and you are back for the annual employer health screen. You step on the scale to get your starting weight because this is the day you take action to change your life. You have a written plan in place not only to eat healthy, but to also address your emotional health as well.

In some cases, you may have a health coach or counselor to help guide you through the process. Keep in mind this is not a temporary change, but a permanent lifestyle change. How many have lost weight to only go back to their old familiar patterns? Long-term success requires caring enough to feed the body and soul with nourishment through healthy food choices and self acceptance. This encourages positive energy flow and harmony.

Taking action is step number four. Today you actively follow a healthy diet and exercise program. It is a challenge, but you are determined to stick with it. Align yourself with positive and supportive people. Avoid those that set out to sabotage your efforts both emotionally and through the dietary changes. It is your life after all. Staying strong, you make it one month, then two, and by the third month you are well on your way to making those bad habits you had a year ago a thing of the past.

The three cans of soda you were drinking a few months ago do not tempt you in the least. You don't even miss them. There are various theories on how long it takes to make a permanent change into a new habit or way of life. My feeling is it generally averages about three months.

You are now well on your way. You feel better and have more energy. The thought of not getting your daily exercise routine in is a source of stress. Three months ago the thought of having to exercise was stressful. You have completely turned around your relationship with food and exercise. The emotional baggage has become much lighter. You are now six months into things and want to maintain and continue on this path of health you are on. Your self-confidence and belief in yourself has been reinforced.

Stage five is all about maintaining and not losing ground and reverting back to bad habits. The positive feedback and change in self-image are motivating you to stay on your path. Stage six is termination. This does not mean you terminate your healthy lifestyle changes. It means that you have been transformed and your goal has been met. A permanent and long-lasting positive change has been made and is now part of who you are (Aschwanden). Congratulations!

You are now not only healthy physically, but emotionally healthy as well. A word of warning needs to be pointed out here however, if you don't address the emotional aspects that contributed to the unhealthy behaviors, there is a high probability you will have to go through this process again. Don't stuff your emotional baggage. Purge it out into the open where you can see it and then heal from it.

The stages of change can be applied to many aspects of our lives. Not just lifestyle changes. Any decision you make often will move through these stages to some degree. Now it may not take a year or more like this example. A change could take seconds, minutes, or days. Not everyone will bring a thought or idea through this whole change process.

The first step to making any change in life is by becoming aware. Without awareness, denial will continue to prevail.

Unhealthy habits will remain and inner peace and fulfillment can remain elusive. Change should not be viewed as a negative. Change means to, *"Challenge Higher Awareness Now to Gain Enlightenment"*. Change is about freeing the body, mind, and soul from dependency to independence.

What we carry around in pounds and emotions is often other peoples' baggage we have allowed to be placed on us. Let it go. Shed it and forget it. There will always be someone ready to judge you. Quit doing what everyone expects you to do. Quit carrying around other people's baggage. You have enough of your own to shed. You can be an angel or a demon and someone will always be judging you. Stop giving up your power. This is your life. Change is about letting go of those things that no longer serve you and taking your power back. Let go of the fear of failure. It is fear that keeps us stuck. Change means releasing the fear and embracing the journey ahead.

So why am I bringing up change now? Why did I not address this at the very beginning? Would you have kept reading? The idea of making a change can stir up negative emotions. I did not want you to see your path to health and healing as something negative. The emotion of fear needs to be replaced with hope. H.O.P.E. means to, *Harness Our Power to Evolve*.

By planting the seeds outlined in the previous chapters you harnessed information on those things that affect your health on many different levels. With the knowledge gained you became more aware of how these factors can also be integrated thereby giving you the power to evolve on your healing path. Every life has meaning and value. To nurture yourself you must first care. I wanted you to care enough to see and once you have seen, change is something you can more readily accept.

There is nothing wrong with whom you are, you just need to *see who you are*. Find the passion and essence of that part of you that you buried by shedding the image of others expectations. It will be transformational. Life will have greater purpose and deeper and richer meaning.

Take Away Tips

- Only you can change you.
- Einstein once said that, "We are boxed in by the boundary conditions of our thinking".
- Fear literally means *Frozen Ego Awaiting Release*
- According to Prochaska's Theoretical Model for Change, there are six stages of change: pre-contemplation, contemplation, preparation, action, maintenance, and termination.
- Change means to: *Challenge Higher Awareness Now to Gain Enlightenment.* Change is about freeing the body, mind, and soul from dependency to independence.
- *HOPE: Harness Our Power to Evolve.*

CHAPTER NINE
Tree of Life

Let's recap what you have learned so far on your path to health and healing. You have gained awareness as to how you can derail your own health. You have also been given tools on how to get back on track to living optimally. You have gained a greater understanding of how stress management, sleep, environment, exercise, diet, and supplements play a pivotal role in changing the quality of our lives. You also understand that when there is an imbalance in any one of these aspects it will affect your gastrointestinal and hormonal health and the body's ability to detoxify properly.

The journey has been an adventure so far and much of what has been discussed are concepts one can grasp on a physical or surface level. These are all concepts that you can see, feel, and consume. Concepts that can sufficiently improve health and one's basic needs such as Maslow refers to as the "Hierarchy of Needs."

There are five levels to Maslow's Hierarchy of Needs. The first of these needs reflect that of basic survival or our physiological needs. We need oxygen, food, water, and sleep in order to survive. When we are born and dependent on our parents, we rely on them to provide the necessities of life. On your path to living a healthier life you may actually stay stuck in these very basic needs of survival when considering changing your diet for example.

If you continue to make poor choices in the foods you consume, your health is likely to deteriorate at a greater rate than the person who takes a more positive view of what changing their diet will mean to their health and well-being and to be the best they can be. They then can move forward to the next level of safety and security. They know changing their lifestyle will be hard, but through the love and support of those around them they gain confidence in their ability to live a healthier life. Their social needs then change as they make a choice to align themselves with people that will support and not try and sabotage their efforts to transform. Through lifestyle changes self-esteem improves and they are now getting closer to the final step of Maslow's Hierarchy of Needs, that of self actualization and being comfortable in their own skin at last (Cherry).

However, to deepen your journey to a whole new level of awareness commands an even broader way of thinking and relating to the world around you. Our lives are full of diverse experiences that impact us not only on a conscious level, but also a subconscious level. The Tree of Life beautifully symbolizes this diversity as a reflection of what not only we see on the surface, but also what is below the surface or that which we can't see.

It is often the subconscious mind that affects the conscious mind and our physical, mental, emotional, and spiritual well-being. By digging down to the roots or the essence of our being we will gain a better understanding of who we are and how we relate to the world around and within. According to the principles of

Traditional Chinese Medicine, that essence, or life force is referred to as *Qi*. It is that invisible energy that permeates every living organism. *Qi* is a reflection of one's physical, mental, emotional, and spiritual health.

Even the great scientist Albert Einstein referred to this energy source as "subtle energy" or that which can't be measured and is the basis of various energy healing modalities (Prout, 18-19). There are an infinite number of paths we can take to healing.

Where is the path you are on leading? What are you striving for? Your tree of life is more than about eating a healthy diet, losing weight, sleeping or starting an exercise routine. It is about even more than Maslow's idea of self-actualization or what motivates us to strive to be our best and to come into who we are as individuals.

That is why the "tree of life" is a symbolic example of self-transformation and our life force. Each one of us is part of something greater. How we relate to each other and the universe as a whole may start out with a simplistic explanation such as Maslow's Hierarchy of Needs. It helps us plant the seed for our own self-transformation and to sprout a beautiful tree of life of health and healing that we can then share and experience with others. The "tree of life" represents knowledge, and through knowledge we gain self awareness and power to see the world from a whole new perspective.

To fully come into our own essence as physical beings we must gain a greater appreciation for our spiritual being as well.

This helps to keep you grounded and to completely transform how you view not only yourself, but the world around you. It means leaving behind the negative aspects that are holding you back, replacing bad *Qi* with good *Qi*.

It means removing the walls or blocks you may have put around you that have kept you from expressing who you are. I think most people believe there is a spiritual presence within and around each of us. We just have to pay attention to it. Prayer is the most common way we tap into the spiritual realm. We are all spiritual beings having a human experience. The karma or baggage we carry with us can impede our health and self-transformation.

I would like you to open your mind and heart to the possibilities of what this means for you. If you are unable to knock down the walls or energy blocks that are holding you back, all the things you have worked on up to this point may increase your chances of slipping back into some of the bad habits you worked so hard to shed. That is where appreciating and accepting your spiritual essence can help you remain on your path to accept and love yourself. If you don't love and accept yourself you cannot fully transform.

There will always be someone in line to judge you. This won't matter when you are fulfilling your purpose and living the life you were meant to live. So many live a life based on the perceived or real expectations of others. Don't hide who you are any longer.

To help open yourself up I think it is helpful to understand that we are all energetic beings. This point can't be argued. Do you want to give off and attract positive or negative energy? If you choose to remain open and positive, that is what you will receive. Negative thoughts will often attract more negative energy. Which do you want to receive? I don't know about you, but I want my light to shine positive.

Learning to tap into positive energy will help protect you from negative forces and surround you with more positive sources of energy. You have free will to make a choice about what it is you want. Make a choice to surround yourself with like-minded individuals that emit positivity.

Now I realize it is human nature to get upset and frustrated sometimes. However, the more you are able to stay grounded in positive ways of thinking, the less often you are likely to be frustrated. You will attract more of what you give off. It is up to you. The energy we give off is a very powerful thing. Dr. Judith Orloff in her book, *Positive Energy*, reflects on this further. There are four laws by which we attract things energetically. Those laws are 1) we attract who we are 2) intuition clarifies smart choices 3) seeing the beauty and goodness in people helps magnetize them 4) and soulful giving generates abundance.

Just reading those four laws of attraction makes you feel better inside, doesn't it?

So what are some of the guiding principles implied within the four laws of energetic attraction? As mentioned, we attract who we are. You get what you give. Love attracts love and anger attracts anger. Staying positive allows you to open your heart to laugh at your imperfections and accept others for theirs. There is no perfect human being. We all have faults and that is what keeps life interesting.

Use your intuition to guide you in the right direction. How many times have you said, "I wish I had listened to my intuition?" This is so important. If something doesn't feel right you will have a physical reaction. Pay attention to it. It may be a sense of uneasiness, a knot in your stomach, or chills or a quiver when things don't feel right. So don't say yes. Say no and walk away. Remove yourself from what doesn't align with your authentic self.

When things do feel right you will be relaxed, open, and at peace. Look for the positive in every situation, even when it doesn't feel right. That is how you continue to grow and blossom. When you say no to someone, it does not have to be a negative. Thank them and move on. If someone is angry, don't get pulled in to the negative energy. Make a conscious decision to turn a negative into a positive. This may mean validating the other person's frustration by stating just that, "I can hear that you are frustrated." This provides validation and can immediately diffuse the situation and clear the air.

If this does not work, you may have to walk away, or ask them to look for a positive solution. Don't look at others' faults, but only at what is good or positive. They may actually be helping you see what you want and don't want for yourself. However, be mindful at the same time not to let others take away your power. Know when it is time to cut the cord and let go of what does not align with your highest good.

Every encounter is an opportunity not to judge ourselves or others, but to learn something about ourselves. This leads to greater openness and giving of our authentic self unconditionally. You will have the capacity to care about other people without expecting anything in return, even when it means cutting the cord. This allows you the capacity to share your greatness, heart and soul (Orloff, 262-284).

So how do I go about opening myself up and working on my emotionally-charged conscious and subconscious blocks? How do I open up and connect more intimately with my spiritual essence or *Qi* to emit and receive this positive energy? How do I keep my light shining, my roots strong and my tree in full bloom?

Emotionally-laden issues will affect our energy centers and can knock us off balance. Eastern philosophy refers to these energy centers as chakras. The chakras align themselves with the nervous, hormonal, and endocrine systems and psychological or emotional areas of the body. Chakras are vibrational energy points that connect with specific organs and emotions. There are seven main chakras. These seven chakras are interconnected so if there is an imbalance or block in one, it can affect the other energy points as well.

Let's look briefly at each of the seven chakras to gain a better understanding of how emotional blocks can affect health and healing.

The first chakra is known as the root chakra. This is what keeps us grounded. This chakra is symbolized by the color red and is located at the base of the spine in the tailbone area. This chakra relates to basic survival and feeling safe and secure. So anything that affects your sense of security and belonging in life can lead to disease in this area. Disease manifestations that can arise from blocks in this area are back problems, arthritis, chronic fatigue, autoimmune disease, and fibromyalgia. It is believed even now by Western medicine that people who suffer from fibromyalgia have experienced some kind of emotional trauma or trigger. Common themes are physical, sexual or emotional abuse or trauma. Other emotional elements affecting this chakra are low self-esteem, shame, guilt, anger, resentment, and unresolved issues.

The second chakra or sacral chakra is located about two inches below the navel area. It is symbolized by the color orange and is associated with what we want, need, and how connected we are in our relationships with others. It is affected by our day-to-day interactions and sense of belonging and feelings of personal and financial security. Sexuality is also very rooted in the second chakra and imbalances in this area can lead to disease and dysfunction in the sexual organs and organs in the pelvic floor including the bladder, appendix, colon, low back, and male and female sex organs.

The third chakra is located in the solar plexus or upper abdomen and symbolized by the color yellow. This area is affected by feelings of self-esteem, self-worth, and self-confidence. Feeling overwhelmed, fearful, inferior, and struggling with responsibilities towards family or your employer can greatly impact this area. How many of you feel like you are not living your life's purpose? Have you ever stopped and asked yourself this question? Are you living to meet everyone else's needs? What is keeping you from believing in yourself? There is an epidemic when it comes to blocks in this area. It seems the whole world has been in turmoil with wars, disease, civil unrest and oppression, job loss, not to mention large cooperation and governmental control and oppression. People are feeling hopeless. This hopelessness manifests as disease and dysfunction of the stomach, intestines, adrenal glands, middle spine, liver, gall bladder, kidneys, pancreas, and esophagus.

How many people do you know that have diabetes, gastric reflux (heartburn), adrenal fatigue, irritable bowel, and fatty liver disease? Probably a more telling question is; do you know anyone that does not have one of these problems?

The fourth chakra is that of the heart and is symbolized by the color green. Green is also known as a healing color. Organs affected by blocks in this area are the heart, lungs, ribs, upper back, shoulders, and breast. Emotional issues in this area include grief, inability to give or receive love, lack of forgiveness, and inability to nurture and care for the self. Self love. If you can't first love yourself, it is difficult to fully give and receive love from others. The blocks in this area may result in conditions such as hypertension, breast problems, heart conditions, asthma, pneumonia, and shoulder problems.

The fifth chakra is that of the throat and symbolized by a sky blue color. This is the point of self expression and communication. Holding back or silencing yourself can result in thyroid disease, neck pain, sore throats, and gum disease. Do you resist voicing your true opinion, thereby silencing yourself?

The sixth chakra is often represented by the color indigo and is often referred to as the third eye. It is located between the eyes. This is the area most commonly associated with intuition, and perception. It is also the area of how we think. Are you rigid and inflexible in your thinking or open and flexible? Do you think rationally or have a knee-jerk reaction to everything? The brain, eyes, ears, nose and pineal gland are affected by blocks in the third eye and may be a factor in learning disabilities, seizure disorders, blindness, deafness, Parkinson's disease, brain tumors, and ringing in the ears.

The seventh or crown chakra is associated with the color purple. It is often referred to as universal source energy or our connection to God. Emotional imbalances here would include not finding your life's purpose, inability to see the larger meaning in life, and how we relate to the world around us, or the lack of a belief system or faith. This does not mean organized religion, but a spiritual belief system that we are connected to something greater than ourselves.

We need to understand that our actions affect the lives of others, not just ourselves. Anything that threatens our existence can lead to blocks in this area and contribute to the manifestation of genetic disorders, multiple sclerosis, developmental disorders, or any number of life-threatening illnesses or accidents (Northrup, 74-97).

So now that you have a better understanding of what can be at the source of emotional and spiritual blocks and physical dysfunction, how do you open those blocks? How do you lessen your chances of disease manifestation? Opening these blocks can help your immune system withstand the emotional interference and clear the energy paths to healing.

Don't blame yourself if you have one of these conditions. There are many factors that can result in the manifestation of disease. Clearing these pathways will help keep you grounded and at peace on an emotional, physical, and spiritual plane. To help us stay grounded, tapping into our chakras or energy source will help keep us open and make our immune systems healthier. There are many studies that have shown how techniques such as meditation can help reduce stress and improve immune function and healing.

This is certainly one way to help open up our chakras. There are many different ways this can be achieved. Certainly applying many of the lifestyle principles discussed is a step in the right direction. However probably even harder than making lifestyle changes are clearing the emotional blocks and being open and accepting of our spiritual beings.

Some methods being used to balance and open our Chakra's you can implement in the privacy of your own home. Others may require the assistance of someone trained in energy healing. Some examples are prayer, meditation, Emotional Freedom Technique (EFT), Theta healing, Quantum touch, Reiki, Healing Touch, Yoga, Tai Chi, and Qigong. A few of these methods were briefly touched on earlier when discussing stress management. It makes sense that if we reduce our stress, our bodies will relax and be more open to healing. It is hard to open blocks on a tired, tense and stressed-out body.

Let's look at some of these methods closer. Some of them are likely familiar to you and others you may not know about. Keep in mind these are only a few of the many energy healing modalities available.

Prayer is one of the easiest and most intimate forms of energy healing. It is our direct line of communication with our spiritual essence to God. It can give us hope when we have none. It may be what keeps you grounded and sane on a daily basis. There have been many studies done to look at the power of prayer and healing. Having worked as a nurse for many years I, like many nurses, have witnessed the power of prayer first-hand.

It can ease the pain and anguish of the sick and dying and their families. I have seen miraculous recoveries that can't be explained by modern medicine. You can actually feel a change in the air and how people relate to each other in the presence of prayer. It is that "subtle energy" Einstein refers to. You can't physically measure it, but you know it is there. It is the conscious act of believing in something greater than ourselves that can hold us up and carry us when we can't do it ourselves.

People have prayed since the beginning of time and have flocked to sacred places praying for a miracle, reporting miracle healings and expressing that they feel they are in a different time or space. Prayer may also be seen as a form of meditation and can help ground us, thereby getting our energy flow back in balance. Whatever you may believe, thought and intent are very powerful. Prayer is a way of holding our intentions and bridging our connections to a Higher Power and to each other.

Meditation, as I mentioned, for some may be a form of prayer and for others, just a state of being present. It is defined as the "process of focusing and concentrating one's attention while maintaining a passive attitude." Many will recite a mantra while meditating, the most common mantra is *OM*. It is believed to create a resonance in the body and that it puts one in touch with a universal energy source.

Meditation helps relax the body and quiet the mind (Dossey, et.al, 574, 577). There are many different forms of meditation. There are formal and informal approaches one can take to meditating. You want to practice a form of meditation that is comfortable to you. It might be as simple as sitting quietly in a room doing breathing exercises or listening to soothing music.

You may meditate with a group of people. Meditation is the quiet in the eye of the storm of our stressed-out and fast-paced lives. Proven health benefits of meditation include stress reduction, emotional healing, inner peace, mental clarity, and life extension (Hyman).

You can find meditations for specific needs such as emotional clearing, stress reduction, healing, and more. There are many aids available to help you with this process. To give you an example, let's look at a meditation that is specific to balancing and clearing your chakras by Anmol Mehta.

Each of the chakra colors will be visualized through this exercise and are considered energy points that connect the physical, mental, and spiritual. Remember that each chakra is located at a particular point along the spine to the crown of the head and that the health of the chakra is reflected by the health of particular organs or regions of the body. By visualizing the color of a particular chakra and through the power of concentration it is believed one can stimulate a particular chakra to open. The chakra colors for your review are

1. Root chakra meditation color: Red
2. Sacral chakra meditation color: Orange
3. Navel chakra meditation color: Yellow
4. Heart chakra meditation color: Green
5. Throat chakra meditation color: Blue
6. Third eye chakra meditation color: Indigo
7. Crown chakra meditation color: Violet

To practice chakra visualization meditation technique, one should follow the step-by-step instructions below.

1. Either lie on your back, or sit up in cross-legged posture with your back straight.
2. Close your eyes and take five deep slow breaths to help relax you and calm the mind.
3. Now begin to visualize the color red at the base of your spine as a glowing ball of red light. Feel your breath moving in and out from this center while continuing to imagine a red ball of light emanating from that location.
4. After spending a minute or two at the root chakra, move up to the sacral chakra and repeat the exercise with the color orange.
5. In this fashion work through all the other chakras as well, where the navel chakra is located at the level of the solar plexus, the heart chakra at the level of the sternum, the throat chakra at the neck and the third eye chakra in the middle of the forehead.
6. Once you complete the cycle, relax for a few minutes and then finish the meditation, by affirming you are healthy, balanced and at peace.

This chakra meditation works through the entire chakra system. You can also focus on opening and balancing just one particular chakra if you have a particular area of concern. Anmol Mehta notes that "this method of chakra balancing is very effective, but one should use it judiciously, as one should be physically able to handle the increased energy flow that can occur when chakras are activated and opened" (Mehta).

Emotional Freedom Technique (EFT) or tapping is a form of psychological acupressure developed by Gary Craig. EFT was born out of the principles of acupuncture and mind-body medicine. It involves tapping common meridian or energy points used by acupuncturists to treat a specific emotional balance.

It is said that negative emotions lead to an imbalance in the body's energy system. EFT involves first tuning into a specific issue and then tapping meridian points with your fingertips. It is believed that EFT when done correctly can help release an emotional issue in minutes or hours as compared to conventional therapy which can take years of work to resolve. Craig states, "EFT can assist physical healing by resolving an underlying emotional cause."

There are five basic steps involved in EFT. First you want to identify an issue. This might be a physical or emotional issue. Be sure to focus on only one issue. You then want to assign intensity to that issue using a one to ten scale with ten being the most intense. This is so you can assess your progress.

For an emotional issue it might involve recreating the memory in your mind. For a physical issue you will note the area of discomfort or pain. The next step is referred to as the "setup." In the setup, you design a phrase or mantra that acknowledges a problem and that you accept yourself in spite of it. For example, at the time of this writing I am experiencing right shoulder pain. So I would want to say, "Even though I have this sore shoulder, I deeply and completely accept myself." You want to address the negative head-on and neutralize it. At the same time you are vocalizing your phrase you will be tapping various meridian points in a specific pattern.

This keeps you tuned in to the issue and stimulates your energy pathways. You sequentially begin by tapping at the top of the head, then at the beginning of the eyebrows, side of the eyes, under the eyes, under the nose, on the chin, at the collar bones, under the arms, and then what is known as the karate chop point at the base of the wrist. You may repeat this sequence as many times as you feel necessary. Then reassess the intensity of your symptoms again. Have they lessened? Maybe even gone? This is just the basic EFT method Craig developed. There are more developed methods that you can learn about or seek out the assistance of someone specifically trained in this technique (Craig).

Theta Healing according to Theta Healing Science and developed by Vianna Stibal, "is essentially applied quantum physics. Using a theta brain wave, which until now was believed to be accessible only in deep sleep or yogi-level meditation, the practitioner is able to connect with the energy of All That Is the energy in everything to identify issues with and witness healings on the physical body, and to identify and change limiting beliefs."

It is literally mind over matter. Research physicists are realizing that the mind can in fact create matter. There is a connection to something greater than us on a deeper spiritual and universal level. Our thoughts create our own reality.

It is believed if you are able to tap into the subconscious beliefs you can change your reality. Theta Healing focuses on prayer and thought. It is believed this helps set the stage for spontaneous healing that conventional medicine can't explain.

Did the person suffering an illness experience a miracle, or through prayer and intent on a subconscious level he or she actually alter reality? I know these are hard concepts to follow. All I can tell you is that if your intent is filled with love, healing can take place. As has been mentioned many times throughout this book, stress is at the root of all disease in the body.

Our perception of the world and how we handle stress is deeply and intimately linked to emotions. If we can replace a negative emotion with positive thoughts and feelings we can clear the subconscious emotional block that is contributing to disease in the physical, mental, emotional and spiritual body (Theta Healing Science).

So how do you tune into the subconscious belief systems? For this it is best to find a practitioner trained in the technique of Theta Healing. A trained practitioner can help you tap into your conscious and subconscious belief systems so you can release emotional blocks. These are often blocks that you are often unaware even exist. The trained Theta Healing practitioner has learned to access theta brain waves while in a conscious state.

Our brains operate at different brain wave levels when we are in different states of consciousness. These include alpha, beta, theta, delta and gamma. The theta brain wave slows down the mind allowing one to access the subconscious mind while being conscious. Theta brain waves are what occur when sleeping and dreaming.

However, you will not be asleep during a Theta Healing session. It is believed this is what healers, mystics and psychics have intuitively been able to do. The brain and the nervous system are very complex and there is so much we don't yet know (Phillips, 1-41). Scientists in the field of psychoneuroimmunology (study of how the mind, nervous and immune systems contribute to disease) and quantum physics are trying to unlock some of these mysteries. So if we can tap into and identify subconsciously held beliefs we can in essence reprogram those limiting beliefs or emotional blocks and potentially change our physical health.

For some of you this concept may be very foreign. For others it will resonate on a deep level. If you are skeptical or don't have access to someone trained in Theta Healing, you can easily purchase theta healing meditation CDs on the internet to try it out. A trained practitioner can guide you to those self limiting beliefs or emotional blocks. This is something you may or may not be able to do on your own.

Quantum Touch, Reiki, and Healing Touch are all forms of energy healing that use the hands, grounding the body and increasing energy flow with the intent to help the body heal itself. Each takes a slightly different approach and the necessary skill to learn these techniques requires various levels of training.

Quantum touch was developed by Richard Gordon. It uses a combination of running energy through the hands and breathing techniques to hold the energy field to promote wellness. Quantum touch is believed to be an effective method for reducing back pain, balancing structural and organ imbalances and aids in healing chronic and acute injuries. This technique is easy to learn, but does require training. There are classes around the country you can attend to learn this technique. You can also seek out the services of someone specifically trained in quantum touch (Quantum Touch).

Reiki is the most widely available form of the energy healing modalities. Reiki was developed by Dr. Mikao Usui in the mid 1800s in Kyoto, Japan. Dr. Usui went on a quest to understand how to heal the body and soul. After searching for many years he felt he discovered the answer to this question from what he learned in the Sanskrit sutras or holy writings, and through consultation with Zen Buddhists, and intense meditation and prayer.

Dr. Usui used symbols from Sanskrit to aid in tuning into *Qi*, the body's Universal Life Energy source, in order to help the body heal itself. Reiki practitioners go through various levels of attunements or degrees of training to tap into the energy and create an environment for healing by placing the hands over or on various parts of the body. Reiki promotes relaxation and stress reduction (J. Morris, Morris, 1-9).

Healing Touch, another form of energy healing, uses the lying on of the hands and was developed by Janet Mentgen in 1989. Janet Mentgen was an energetically-sensitive nurse who recognized how powerful touch was in helping patients and began to hone her skills energetically. Healing Touch practitioners, like the other hands-on healing modalities, goes through a series of levels of training. Healing Touch training requires a more intensive training and is only available to those people that already have training in the health sciences such as a nurse, physician, massage therapist, psychotherapist, counselor, and other health professionals.

All these healing energies keep in mind a focus on intent and Universal love. The Healing Touch practitioner uses his or her hands to hold the energy field that surrounds the body to help facilitate physical, emotional, and spiritual health and healing.

All three of the forms of hands-on healing discussed have research to support their validity. Healing Touch has the most scientifically-based research and scientists are beginning to realize that something is happening when energy healing is used. Healing Touch studies have been conducted in hospitals, universities, private organizations, the National Institutes of Health, and other reputable places. All support the notion that Healing Touch has benefit. Even if you don't believe in such things, which I hope you do, these energy healing modalities are noninvasive, economical, and beneficial (Healing Touch Program).

When discussing the various forms of energy healing up to this point, most of these have required specific training and the assistance of a practitioner to assist you in tapping into the energy field to aid self healing. But what if this is not an option for you? You might not have access to an energy healing practitioner or maybe you can't afford the treatments.

Unfortunately insurance does not reimburse for these types of treatments. This is a shame in a world where we have out-of-control health care costs. Work with an energy practitioner is a fraction of what it would cost to take a pill box full of medications along with their potential side effects. Don't get me wrong, there is a time and place for medications and many are necessary.

The problem is that a pill is not going to fix everything. A pill is not going to fix the physical, mental, and emotional imbalance that have their roots in conscious and subconscious stress and emotion. Did I not say that stress is at the very core of all disease? Energy healing is aimed to help the body to relax and heal. If the body is put into a state of relaxation, various negative physiological patterns that occur with stress will be reduced and a more healing physiological pattern will take over. The body has an enormous capacity to heal itself if we let it.

So what can you do, either on your own or in a class setting, to support relaxation and reduce stress? There are three forms of exercise that almost anyone can do that will help with stress reduction, increase strength and flexibility and support immune function. I am talking about Yoga, Tai Chi, and Qigong.

All three are intended to connect the mind, body, and spirit through a series of movements and breathing.

Early Yoga dates back more than 5,000 years and was used for physical and mental exercise. Yoga, through breathing, meditation and exercise is designed to put pressure on the glandular systems of the body to support healing. Yoga involves a series of stretching exercises and postures. There are many different forms of yoga that one can practice. You want to find one that resonates with you.

Tai Chi is an ancient Chinese exercise. The person doing Tai Chi will go through a series of dance-like movement in a smooth and continuous fashion. This aids in helping the individual with concentration, strengthening and relaxation. In the elderly it has been shown to help improve balance and posture (Dossey, et.al., 273-274). Like Tai Chi, Qigong's roots can be traced back more than 4,000 years to China. Qigong literally means energy practice or cultivating the body's vital energy so the body can strengthen and heal. Qigong exercise is a form of rhythmic meditation and deep breathing connecting the mind, body, and spirit. It is believed to help open up the meridians or energy pathways of the body. It is becoming increasingly popular in the United States as people are on a quest for more natural ways of health and healing.

In 2007 it was estimated that 625,000 Americans were regularly practicing Qigong. Studies have shown that Qigong can help in relieving the symptoms of fibromyalgia, Parkinson's, arthritis, depression, hypertension, and diabetes (Qi Gong). All three forms of energy movement and exercise are growing in popularity and have health benefits.

As you can see, there are many paths you can take on your quest to health and healing. Health is not just about eating a healthy diet and getting regular exercise, but more importantly it is a state of mind. How great our health care system would be if all levels of knowledge that Western Medicine, (the trunk or what you can see), and Eastern Medicine, (the roots, or what you can't see) were brought together?

There are many health care providers who are on this path, for example those that actively practice Integrative and Functional Medicine. Unfortunately their practices have often come under attack from their own colleagues, the media, and our government.

But I think there is an enormous shift taking place. People are demanding more from their health care and are challenging their health care providers as more information than ever before can be found by searching the Internet. You know there is more to your health than a symptom and we are demanding more answers. Many conventional trained health care providers have made a choice just as you have made a choice to demand more answers. Some health care providers will turn a blind eye to this information and will immediately discount it without finding the research to support their biased opinion. Others will listen and look for research that supports a given claim you may present them with.

Much of the research that supports a more holistic approach is sadly not often found in traditional medical journals that are largely supported by pharmaceutical companies and advertisements for medicines.

There are some very good scientifically-based alternative medical journals to which only a small number of providers subscribe. However, as public demand for a more integrative approach to care continues to grow, and in order for conventional medicine to keep up, they are going to need to open their hearts and minds or they will be left behind. I truly believe that most of us that got into health care did so because we felt a calling to help others as part of our life purpose.

In defense of conventional medicine, the pressure to run you through an assembly line is the only way they can stay afloat due to poor reimbursement, governmental regulations, and the overhead cost of running the business of health care.

Many of those who have chosen to take the path of integrative and functional medicine do not take insurance, thereby eliminating many of these issues and allowing them to spend more time with their patients and to stop and listen to you the patient. The therapeutic value of this can't be understated. At the time of the writing of this book there is talk of paying or reimbursing providers for the quality of care they provide, not the quantity of patients. I hope this is true, for there should be a greater emphasis on helping you to address root causes along your path to health and healing.

Take Away Tips

- Maslow's Five Hierarchy of Needs: physiological, safety, love and belonging, esteem, and self-actualization.
- The Tree of Life beautifully symbolizes the diversity as a reflection of what not only we see on the surface, but also what is below the surface -or that which we can't see.
- The Tree of Life is a symbolic example of self transformation.
- *Qi* is the invisible energy that permeates every living organism.
- There are many ways to help clear emotional blocks including opening your chakras, prayer, meditation, energy healing, and meditative exercise.

CHAPTER TEN
Transformation

I am honored that you have taken the time to read this book. My life, like yours, is all about transformation. Transformation is about changing those things that no longer serve us. In order to transform you first must become aware that there is a problem. You can't transform a weakened and tangled root system if you don't see the mess in the first place. Ignoring what is right in front of you or blaming someone else or even yourself does not help. The past is the past. Be present in the now, leave the tangled mess behind and start to nourish your roots in a positive and loving manner. Now that you are aware and are about to embark on a clearer path, start moving forward one step at a time.

We all are faced with many choices every day. Each of us will be faced with many challenges in life. Those challenges shape who we are and what we may become. The way we choose to respond to those challenges can have a profound impact on our health. As I mentioned early on, you don't have to resign yourself to the fate of your parents or grandparents when it comes to your health. If they had diabetes, heart disease, cancer, depression, does that mean you have to give up? Do you say, I am going to live life to the fullest with a poor diet, lack of exercise, smoking, and/or alcohol, because I am going to end up getting one of these diseases, just like my parents and their parents? I hope not.

As you learned in this book, your genetics are only one small part of the equation. The lifestyle choices you make have a much greater impact. I refuse to accept the notion that I will get heart disease like my father, or diabetes like my mother. I have chosen instead to use every day to work on the very principles I have presented to you. Am I perfect? Absolutely not, but the vast majority of the time I have chosen to eat a healthy diet, exercise, get adequate sleep and try to limit the stressors in my life. The key word here is chosen. So I hope you will choose wisely as you explore your own self-transformation.

Transformation is the process of constant change. We are always evolving and must be flexible to try new things, face our fears, opening our hearts and minds, and feeling our emotions. Like the roots of a tree, our life and how we choose to live it, is affected by a complex network of physical, emotional, environment, and spiritual factors.

Part of transforming this network is taking responsibility for yourself and learning to love who you are as a person. Loving who you are and being what you are meant to be will free you from the constraints you or those constraints you have allowed society to place on you start to disappear. This can be a very freeing experience and will make any burdens you carry feel lighter.

The path to transforming your health will likely be met with some fear and resistance. Face your fears head-on. Start knocking down those emotional blocks that are keeping you stuck. You have the capacity to experience a life of abundance and healing. Your life is what you choose to make of it, no excuses. Only through love and acceptance can you transform your destiny. Only through love can you connect the best of your mind, body, and spirit in ways you never dreamt possible.

By connecting to the spiritual essence of who you are and Universal love or God we can find our way home. Just like Dorothy in the *"Wizard of Oz,"* close your eyes, click your heels three times and you too can find your way home to who you truly are. Feel with your heart more and with your head less. Ego will block your higher awareness and personal transformation. Think of transformation as something positive as I share one last acronym to leave you with. Transformation means: *Turn Resistance Away Now So Freeing Options Reveal Many Avenues To Infiniteness Of Nirvana*. Nirvana means to be free of mind, body, and spirit and free of suffering. Be free to find your own peace within.

In closing, I would like to share this quote from Sonia Choquette from her book, *Vitamins for the Soul,* titled *Align Yourself with the Universe*. "When you expect your Higher Self to guide you, you place your full attention, both conscious and subconscious, directly on your Higher Self. This shifts your attention from other people trying to run your life, and places your power in the hands of the Divine. By making this decision, you become a person who responds to life, rather than one who reacts to it. Expecting Divine assistance realigns you with God and the Universe at all times. Trusting your vibes to guide you will help you attract all you need to succeed." (45).

These are wonderful and divinely inspired words to live by. God bless you on your journey and your path to health and healing.

Recommended Readings

Braverman, Eric R. *Younger You: Unlock the Hidden Power of Your Brain to Look and Feel 15 Years Younger.* New York: McGraw-Hill, 2007. Print.

Campbell, T. *The China Study, The Most Comprehensive Study of Nutrition Ever Conducted.* Dallas, TX: Benbella, 2006. Print.

Dale, Theresa. *Revitalize Your Hormones: Dr. Dale's 7 Steps to a Happier, Healthier, and Sexier You.* Hoboken, NJ: John Wiley, 2005. Print.

Feinstein, Alice. *Nutri-cures: Foods & Supplements That Work with Your Body to Relieve Symptoms & Speed Healing.* New York, NY: Rodale, 2010. Print.

Faloon, William. *Pharmocracy: How Corrupt Deals and Misguided Medical Regulations Are Bankrupting America-- and What to Do about It.* Mount Jackson, VA: Praktikos, 2011. Print.

Gittleman, Ann Louise. *Zapped: Why Your Cell Phone Shouldn't Be Your Alarm Clock and 1,268 Ways to Outsmart the Hazards of Electronic Pollution.* New York: Harper One, 2010. Print.

Goodman, Myra, Linda Holland, and Pamela McKinstry. *Food to Live By: The Earthbound Farm Organic Cookbook.* New York: Workman Pub., 2006. Print.

Hyman, Mark, and Donna Boland. *The Ultrametabolism Cookbook: 200 Delicious Recipes That Will Turn on Your Fat-burning DNA*. New York: Scribner, 2007. Print.

Hyman, Mark M. D. *The UltraMind Solution*. New York, NY: Scribner, 2009. Print.

Lucille, Holly. *Creating and Maintaining Balance: A Woman's Guide to Safe, Natural Hormone Health*. Boulder, CO: IMPAKT/Health, 2004. Print.

Mindell, Earl, and Virginia Hopkins. *Prescription Alternatives: Hundreds of Safe, Natural, Prescription-free Remedies to Restore & Maintain Your Health*. New York: McGraw-Hill, 2009. Print.

Northrup, Christiane. *Women's Bodies, Women's Wisdom: Creating Physical and Emotional Health and Healing*. Third ed. New York: Bantam, 2006. Print.

Orloff, Judith. *Positive Energy: 10 Extraordinary Prescriptions for Transforming Fatigue, Stress, and Fear into Vibrance, Strength, and Love*. New York: Harmony, 2004. Print.

Somers, Suzanne. *Bombshell: Explosive Medical Secrets That Will Redefine Aging*. New York: Crown Archetype, 2012. Print.

Somers, Suzanne. *Knockout: Interviews with Doctors Who Are Curing Cancer and How to Prevent Getting It in the First Place*. First ed. New York: Crown, 2009. Print.

Taylor, Pamela L. *Simple Ways of Healing: A Textbook of Natural Therapies*. First ed. Moline, IL: MidWest Botanicals, LLC, 2007. Print.

Teitelbaum, Jacob. *From Fatigued to Fantastic!: A Clinically Proven Program to Regain Vibrant Health and Overcome Chronic Fatigue and Fibromyalgia*. Third ed. New York: Avery, 2007. Print.

Timmins, William G. *The Chronic Stress Crisis: How Stress Is Destroying Your Health and What You Can Do to Stop It*. Bloomington, IN: AuthorHouse, 2009. Print.

Weil, Andrew. *Eating Well for Optimum Health: The Essential Guide to Food, Diet, and Nutrition*. New York: Knopf, 2000. Print.

Weil, Andrew. *Spontaneous Healing: How to Discover and Enhance Your Body's Natural Ability to Maintain and Heal Itself*. New York: Knopf, 1995. Print.

References

Chapter 1: Planting the Seed

"Institute for Functional Medicine What Is Functional Medicine?" *Institute for Functional Medicine What Is Functional Medicine?* N.p., n.d. Web. 14 Jan. 2012. <http://www.functionalmedicine.org/about/whatisfm/>.

Chapter 2: Sleep

Belsky, G. "Potential Sleep Saboteurs: 8 Factors That Could Be Keeping You Awake at Night." *Http://www.health.com/health/condition-article/0,,20188024,00.html*. N.p., 06 May 2008. Web. 01 Feb. 2012.

Colten, H., and B. Altevogt. "SLEEP DISORDERS AND SLEEP DEPRIVATION." *Sleep Disorders and Sleep Deprivation: An Unmet Public Health Problem*. N.p., n.d. Web. 20 Jan. 2012. <http://www.nap.edu/openbook.php?record_id=11617>.

"Everyday Oils." *Young Living Essential Oils*. N.p., n.d. Web. 21 Jan. 2012. <https://www.youngliving.org/oils4wellness>.

"Getting the Recommended Amounts of Key Nutrients, Maintaining a Healthy Weight and Eating a Heart Healthy Diet Is Essential for Good Health." *Importance of Sleep : Six Reasons Not to Scrimp on Sleep*. N.p., Jan. 2006. Web. 21 Jan. 2012.

<http://www.health.harvard.edu/press_releases/importance_of_sleep_and_health>.

Hyman, Mark M. D. *The UltraMind Solution*. New York, NY: Scribner, 2009. 169. Print.

"NINDS Narcolepsy Information Page." *Narcolepsy Information Page: National Institute of Neurological Disorders and Stroke (NINDS)*. N.p., n.d. Web. 21 Jan. 2012. <http://www.ninds.nih.gov/disorders/narcolepsy/narcolepsy.htm>.

"Importance of Sleep: Six Reasons Not to Scrimp on Sleep." *Harvard Health Publications* (Jan. 2006): *Health.Harvard.edu*. Web. 20 Jan. 2012. <http://www.health.harvard.edu/press_releases/importance_of_sleep_and_health>.

Staff, Mayo Clinic. "Definition." *Mayo Clinic*. Mayo Foundation for Medical Education and Research, 19 Jan. 2012. Web. 20 Jan. 2012. <http://www.mayoclinic.com/health/restless-legs-syndrome/DS00191/METHOD=print>.

Stevens, S., and S. Benbadis. "Normal Sleep, Sleep Physiology, and Sleep Deprivation ." *Normal Sleep, Sleep Physiology, and Sleep Deprivation*. N.p., 05 Dec. 2011. Web. 20 Jan. 2012. <http://emedicine.medscape.com/article/1188226-overview>.

Talbott, Shawn. *The Cortisol Connection*. Second ed. Alameda, CA: Hunter House, 2007. 96+. Print.

Teitelbaum, Jacob. *From Fatigued to Fantastic!: A Clinically Proven Program to Regain Vibrant Health and Overcome Chronic Fatigue and Fibromyalgia*. Third ed. New York: Avery, 2007. 49-52. Print.

Chapter 3: Environment

American Lung Associate. *American Lung Association Report Highlights Toxic Health Threat of Coal-Fired Power Plants, Calls for the EPA to Reduce Emissions and Save Lives*. N.p., 08 May 2011. Web. 29 Jan. 2012. <http://www.lung.org/press-room/press-releases/power-plants-epa.html>.

Brockovich, Erin. "Erin Brockovich Biography." *Erin Brockovich Biography*. N.p., n.d. Web. 28 Jan. 2012. <http://www.brockovich.com/mystory.html>.

Environmental Protection Agency. *Our Mission and What We Do*. N.p., n.d. Web. 28 Jan. 2012. <http://www.epa.gov/aboutepa/whatwedo.html>.

Environmental Protection Agency. *What Is Acid Rain?* N.p., n.d. Web. 28 Jan. 2012. <http://www.epa.gov/acidrain/what/index.html>.

"Fluoride Chloride DRI/RDA, Benefits, Side Effects, Overdose, Toxicity, Requirements." *Fluoride Chloride DRI/RDA, Benefits, Side Effects, Overdose, Toxicity, Requirements*. N.p., n.d. Web. 28 Jan. 2012. <http://www.acu-cell.com/fcl.html>.

Fuch, N. "Filters Can't Protect You From Toxic Water but This Can." *Women's Health Letter* 17.9 (2011): 1-3. Print.

Fuchs, N. "Are You Rubbing Poison on Your Skin?" *Women's Health Letter* (2010): n. pag. Print.

Fuchs, N. "How Electropullution Zaps Your Health and Causes Chronic Illness." *Women's Health Letter* 17(2) (2011): 1-4. Print.

Fuchs, N. "The Overlooked Pollution That Can Ruin Your Health and How to Protect Yourself." *Women's Health Letter* 17(1) (2011): 1-3. Print.

Gittleman, Ann Louise. *Zapped: Why Your Cell Phone Shouldn't Be Your Alarm Clock and 1,268 Ways to Outsmart the Hazards of Electronic Pollution.* New York: Harper One, 2010. Print.

Bland, Jeffrey S. *Textbook of Functional Medicine.* Third ed. Gig Harbor, WA.: Institute for Functional Medicine, 2010. 147-50. Print.

Mercola, Dr. Joseph. "The Health Hazards of Water Fluoridation (VIDEO)." *The Huffington Post.* TheHuffingtonPost.com, 11 Oct. 2010. Web. 29 Jan. 2012. <http://www.huffingtonpost.com/dr-mercola/warning-this-daily-habit-_b_741635.html>.

"Multi-Center Study Shows Direct Link Between Residential Radon Exposure and Lung Cancer." *ScienceDaily.* ScienceDaily, 08 Apr. 2005. Web. 21 Mar. 2012. <http://www.sciencedaily.com/articles/r/radon.htm>.

Weil, Andrew. *Spontaneous Healing: How to Discover and Enhance Your Body's Natural Ability to Maintain and Heal Itself.* New York: Knopf, 1995. 157-61. Print.

World Health Organization. *What Are Electromagnetic Fields?* N.p., n.d. Web. 04 Feb. 2012. <http://www.who.int/peh-emf/about/WhatisEMF/en/>.

World Health Organization. *WHO.* N.p., n.d. Web. 28 Jan. 2012. <http://www.who.int/topics/environmental_health/en/>.

Yu, Wih-Ru. "Pesticides and Parkinson' Disease." *Acta Neurologica Taiwanica* 14.2 (2005): 38-39. Print.

Chapter 4: Exercise

Abdo, J. "Creating Ourselves." *LifeExtension.com.* N.p., Apr. 1998. Web. 11 Feb. 2012. <http://www.lef.org/magazine/mag98/apr98fitness.htm?.>.

De Gonzalez, B., A. Hartge, and P. Cerhand, JR. "Body-Mass Index and Mortality among White Adults." *New England Journal of Medicine* 363.23 (2010): 2211-219. Print.

Faloon, W. "An Epidemic of Denial." *Life Extension* July 2011: 7-14. Web. <http://www.lef.org/>.

Goepp, J. "Critical Need for Multi-Modal Approach to Combat Obesity." *Life Extension* June 2009: 27-35. Web.

Hyman, Mark M. D. *The UltraMind Solution.* New York, NY: Scribner, 2009. 314-15. Print.

Musnick, David. "Clinical Approaches to Structural Imbalance." *Textbook of Functional Medicine*. Third ed. Gig Harbor: Institute of Functional Medicine, 2010. 481-87. Print.

Smith, J., T. Sheets, and S. Watson. "Is There More to Yoga than Exercise?" *Alternative Therapies* 17.3 (2011): 22-29. Print.

Talbott, Shawn M. *The Cortisol Connection: Why Stress Makes You Fat and Ruins Your Health and What You Can Do about It*. Second ed. Alameda, CA: Hunter House, 2007. 145. Print.

Wood, Layne. "What Are the Benefits of Yoga & Pilates?" *LIVESTRONG.COM*. N.p., 15 Jan. 2011. Web. 11 Feb. 2012. <http://www.livestrong.com/article/357590-what-are-the-benefits-of-yoga-pilates/>.

Chapter 5: Diet

Campbell, T. "Eating Right: Eight Principles of Food and Health." *The China Study, The Most Comprehensive Study of Nutrition Ever Conducted*. By T. Campbell. Dallas, TX: Benbella, 2006. 225-40. Print.

De Lorgeril, M., P. Salen, I. Monjaud, J. Delaye, and N. Mamell. "Mediterranean Diet, Traditional Risk Factors, and the Rate of Cardiovascular Complications after Myocardial Infarction: Final Report of the Lyon Diet Heart Study."
Circulation 99.6 (1999): 779-85. Print.

Fife, Bruce. *Coconut Cures: Preventing and Treating Common Health Problems with Coconut.* Colorado Springs, CO: Piccadilly, 2005. 6-56. Print.

"Doctor Oz." *GMO Foods: Are They Dangerous to Your Health?* CBS. New York, New York, 17 Oct. 2012. Television.

"Glycemic Index: Making Healthy Choices Easy." The University of Sydney, Glycemic Index Foundation, n.d. Web. 19 Feb. 2012. <http://www.glycemicindex.com/>.

Hyman, M. "Three Hidden Ways Wheat Makes You Fat." *The UltraWellness Center of Mark Hyman, MD*. N.p., n.d. Web. 19 Feb. 2012. <http://www.ultrawellnesscenter.com/2012/02/13/three-hidden-ways-wheat-makes-you-fat/>.

Kastorini, C., H. Milionis, K. Esposito, D. Guigliano, J. Goudevenos, and D. Panagiotakos. "The Effect of Mediterranean Diet on Metabolic Syndrome and Its Components." *Journal of the American College of Cardiology* 57.11 (2011): 1299-313. Print.

"Mediterranean Diet & Pyramid." *Oldways Preservation Trust*. N.p., n.d. Web. 26 Feb. 2012. <http://www.oldwayspt.org/resources/heritage-pyramids/mediterranean-diet-pyramid>.

Staff, Mayo Clinic. "Mediterranean Diet: Choose This Heart-healthy Diet Option." *Mayo Clinic*. Mayo Foundation for Medical Education and Research, 19 June 2010. Web. 18 Feb. 2012.

<https://www.mayoclinic.com/health/mediterranean-diet/CL00011>.

State of Science Review. *New Evidence Confirms the Nutritional Superiority of Plant-based Organic Foods.* By C. Benbrook, X. Zhao, J. Yanez, N. Davies, and P. Andrews. Organiccenter.org, Mar. 2008. Web. 26 Feb. 2012. <http://www.organic-center.org/science.nutri.php?action=view>.

United Nations Educational, Scientific and Cultural Organization. *Mediterranean Diet.* N.p., 2010. Web. 18 Feb. 2012. <http://www.unesco.org/culture/ich/index.php?lg=en>.

Chapter 6: Supplements

Allen, D. *Essential Oil Research Report, Weber University.* Rep. N.p., Sept. 1997. Web. 07 Mar. 2012. <http://www.webdeb.com/studies.htm>.

"Archives." *Homeopathic Research.* N.p., n.d. Web. 08 Mar. 2012. <http://www.homeopathy.org/portfolio_category/homeopathic-research/>.

"Botanicals." *Gale Encyclopedia of Food & Culture.* N.p., n.d. Web. 08 Sept. 2012. <http://www.answers.com/topic/botanical>.

Clement, Brian. "Killer Fish." *Healing Our World* Sept. 2012: 17+. Web. <http://www.hippocrateshealthinstitute.org>.

Complementary Alternative Cancer TherapiesCancer Patient Nutrition Therapies. *LifeExtension.org*. N.p., 2009. Web. 06 Mar. 2012. http://www.lef.org/protocols/cancer/alternative_cancer_therapies_01.htm?source=search>.

Dale, T. "Homeopathy." *Wellnesscenter.net*. N.p., n.d. Web. 15 Mar. 2011. <http://www.wellnesscenter.net/resources/articles/Homeopathy_Description.htm>.

Dale, Theresa. "Powerful Hormone Revitalization with Homeopathy." *Revitalize Your Hormones: Dr. Dale's 7 Steps to a Happier, Healthier, and Sexier You*. Hoboken, NJ: John Wiley, 2005. 188-202. Print.

DaVanoz, D., S. Heath, and A. Dobson. "The Economic Contribution of the Dietary Supplement Industry: Analyses of the Economic Benefits to the U.S. Economy." *Natural Products Foundation | Natural Products Foundation*. N.p., May 2009. Web. 06 Mar. 2012. <http://www.naturalproductsfoundation.org/index.php?src=gendocs>.

Deardorff, Julie. "Homeopathy Prospers Even as Controversy Rages." *Phys.org*. N.p., 11 Mar. 2011. Web. 17 Mar. 2012. <http://phys.org/news/2011-03-homeopathy-prospers-controversy-rages.html>.

Ehrlich, S. "Calcium Overview." *University of Maryland Medical*

Center. N.p., 2011. Web. 07 Mar. 2012. <http://www.umm.edu/altmed/articles/calcium-000290.htm>.

"Everyday Oils." *Young Living*. N.p., n.d. Web. 07 Mar. 2012. <http://www.youngliving.com/essential-oil-collections/Everyday-Oils>.

Fisher, Tom. "The 1-2-3s of Omega-3s." *Healing Our World* Sept. 2012: 19+. Web. <http://hippocrateshealthinstitue.org>.

Frenkel, M., B. Mishra, and P. Yang. "Cytotoxic Effects of Ultra-diluted Remedies on Breast Cancer Cells." *International Journal of Oncology* 36 (2009): 395-403. Print.

Jegtvig, S. "Dietary Supplements." *Www.about.com*. N.p., n.d. Web. 06 Mar. 2012. <http://nutrition.about.com/od/nutrition101/ss/healthy_new_yea_4.htm>.

Killian, J. "The Overlooked Role of Probiotics in Human Health." *Life Extension* Apr. 2012: 29-39. Print.

Mehta, Bella, and Carol Rollins. "OTC Advisor: Popular Herbal and Dietary Supplements." Lecture. American Pharmacists Association, 30 July 2010. Web. 06 Mar. 2010. <http://elearning.pharmacist.com/Portal/Files/LearningProducts/7bd326737b644fd28966ed5def2ef7fb/assets/037_OTC%20ADV_Herbal%20and%20Dietary%20Supplements_New%20Final%20072910.pdf>.

Mercola, J. ""Still Taking Fish Oil? Check Out This New Warning..."" *Mercola.com*. N.p., n.d., Web. 09 Mar. 2012. <http://krilloil.mercola.com/krill-oil.html>.

Montagnier, L. "French Nobelist Escapes Intellectual Terror to Pursue Radical Ideas in China." *Science* 330 (2010): 1732. Print.

Mullin, Gerard E., and Kathie Madonna. Swift. "Supplements to Health your Inside Tract." *The Inside Tract: Your Good Gut Guide to Great Digestive Health*. New York, NY: Rodale, 2011. 149-50. Print.

National Center for Complimentary and Alternative Medicine. *Are You considering Cam?* Nccam.nih.gov, 2006. Web. 06 Mar. 2012. <http://nccam.nih.gov/health/decisions/consideringcam.htm>.

National Center for Disease Control and Prevention. *Drug-Induced Deaths--United States, 2003-2007*. By L. Paulozzi. Cdc.gov, 14 Jan. 2011. Web. 06 Mar. 2012. <http://www.cdc.gov/mmwr/preview/mmwrhtml/su6001a12.htm>.

National Institutes of Health. Office of Dietary Supplements. *Botanical Dietary Supplements: What Is a Botanical?* N.p., n.d. Web. 07 Mar. 2012. <http://ods.od.nih.gov/factsheets/BotanicalBackground-HealthProfessional/>.

National Institutes of Health. Office of Dietary Supplements.

    Dietary Supplement Fact Sheet: Calcium. N.p., n.d. Web.

    07 Mar. 2012. <htt://ods.od.nih.gov/factsheets/calcium/>.

Pick, M. "Gut Flora on a Crusade for Good." *Advance for NP's &*

    Pa's 3.3 (2012): 35-36. Print.

Prabuseenivasan, S., M. Jayakumar, and S. Ignacimuthu. "In Vitro

    Antibacterial Activity of Some Plant Essential Oils."

Biomed Central Complimentary and Alternative Medicine

    6.39 (2006): 1-8. Print.

Rowen, Robert. "The One Chlorella Product I Trust More than

    Any Other." *Advancedbionutritionals.com.* N.p., n.d. Web.

    20 Apr. 2012. <http://www.advancedbionutritionals.com/

    Products/King-Chlorella.htm>.

Saul, Andrew W. "Doctor Yourself: An Interview with Andrew W.

    Saul." *Innerexplorations.com.* N.p., n.d. Web. 06 Mar.

    2012. <http://www.innerexplorations.com/

    simpletext/andrew.htm>.

Shumway, D., G. Maskarinec, H. Kakai, and C. Gotay. "Why

    Some Cancer Patients Choose Complimentary and

    Alternative Medicine Instead of Conventional Treatment."

    (n.d.): n. pag. *The Journal of Family Practice.* Dec. 2001.

    Web. 07 Mar. 2012. <http://www.jfponline.com/

    Pages.asp?AID=2399&issue=December 2001&UID=>.

Smith, Philip. "Michael F. Holick, PhD, MD the Pioneer of Vitamin D Research." *Life Extension* 1 Sept. 2010: 52-57. Print.

Stengler, Mark. "Tumeric." *The Natural Physician's Healing Therapies: Proven Remedies That Medical Doctors Don't Know about*. Stamford, CT: Bottom Line, 2007. 444-46. Print.

"Vitamin D." *Natural Standard - Restricted Access Login*. N.p., 2012. Web. 08 Mar. 2012. <http://naturalstandard.com/databases/refs-vitamind.asp>.

"Vitamins, Minerals and Supplements." *Guide*. N.p., n.d. Web. 09 Mar. 2012. <http://www.vitaguide.org/>.

Vitamins. U.S. National Library of Medicine, n.d. Web. 09 Mar. 2012. <http://www.nlm.nih.gov/medlineplus/ency/article/002399.htm>.

Watson, B. *The H.O.P.E. Formula: The Ultimate Health Secret*. N.p.: Renew Life and Information Services, 2006. 60-61. Print.

"What Are Essential Oils?" *Essential Oil University*. N.p., n.d. Web. 07 Mar. 2012. <http://essentialoils.org/>.

Chapter 7: Four undiscovered pathways to health

Bland, J. "Environmental Inputs." *Textbook of Functional Medicine*. Third ed. Gig Harbor: Institute of Functional Medicine, n.d. 138-40. Print.

Bowden, J. "Get Rid of Candida for Good!" *Total Health Breakthroughs: Alternative Solutions for Mind, Body, and Soul* (03 July 2009): n. pag. *Total Health Breakthroughs.* Web. 04 Apr. 2012. <http://www.totalhealthbreakthroughs.com/author/dr-jonny-bowden/>.

Braverman, Eric R. *Younger You: Unlock the Hidden Power of Your Brain to Look and Feel 15 Years Younger.* New York: McGraw-Hill, 2007. Print.

Dale, T. "Homeopathy." *Menopause Symptoms, Women's Health, Education, Naturopathy, Saliva Test.* N.p., n.d. Web. 15 Mar. 2011. <http://www.wellnesscenter.net/resources/articles/Homeopathy_Description.htm>.

Dale, Theresa. "Emotional-Management Techniques for Inner Revitalization." *Revitalize Your Hormones: Dr. Dale's 7 Steps to a Happier, Healthier, and Sexier You.* Hoboken, NJ: John Wiley, 2005. 169-77. Print.

Davis, Reed. "Steroidal Hormone Principal Pathways." *Functional Diagnostic Nutrition RSS.* N.p., n.d. Web. 15 Dec. 2012.

Frenkel, M., B. Mishra, S. Sen, and P. Yang. "Cytotoxic Effects of Ultra-diluted Remedies on Breast Cancer Cells." *International Journal of Oncology* 36.2 (2009): 395-403. Print.

"Function of the Intestinal Barrier." *BioHealth Diagnostics.* N.p., n.d. Web. 31 Mar. 2012. <http://intestinalbarriertest.com/pdf/Function-Intestinal-Barrier.pdf>.

Galland, Leo, and Helen Lafferty. "Flora, Intestinal Permeability, and Immune Response." *Gastrointestinal Dysregulation: Connections to Chronic Disease*. Gig Harbor, WA: Institute for Functional Medicine, 2008. 25-32. Print.

Hirashiki, J. "Banish Fatigue, Enhance Gratitude and Take Responsibility." *Health Keepers* December.29 (2011): 36-37. Print.

Hyman, M. "Gluten: What You Don't Know Might Kill You." *Huffington Post*. N.p., 02 Jan. 2010. Web. 31 Mar. 2012. <http://www.huffingtonpost.com/dr-mark-hyman/gluten-what-you-dont-know_b_379089.html?>.

Lee, John R., and Virginia Hopkins. "What Is Estrogen?" *What Your Doctor May Not Tell You about Menopause: The Breakthrough Book on Natural Progesterone*. New York, NY: Warner, 1996. 34-43. Print.

Liska, D. "Influence of Mind and Spirit." *Textbook of Functional Medicine*. Third ed. Gig Harbor, WA.: Institute for Functional Medicine, 2005. 165-66. Print.

Lorentz, M. "Stress and Psychoneuroimmunology Revisited: Using Mind-body Interventions to Reduce Stress." *Alternative Journal of Nursing* July.11 (2006): 1-6. Print.

Lucille, Holly. "Addressing the Underlying Cause." *Creating and Maintaining Balance: A Woman's Guide to Safe, Natural Hormone Health*. Boulder, CO: IMPAKT/Health, 2004. 23-25. Print.

Lucille, Holly. "The Stress Connection." *Creating and Maintaining Balance: A Woman's Guide to Safe, Natural Hormone Health.* Boulder, CO: IMPAKT/Health, 2004. 66-67. Print.

McEvoy, M. "The Endocrine Journey: Steroidal Hormones & Their Pathways." *Metabolichealing.com.* N.p., 12 Jan. 2012. Web. 14 Apr. 2012. <http://metabolichealing.com/key-integrated-functions-of-your-body/hormone-and-endocrine/the-endocrine-journey-steroidal-hormones-and-their-pathways/>.

Mullin, Gerard E., and Kathie Madonna. Swift. "The "Inside Tract" to a Better Health." *The Inside Tract: Your Good Gut Guide to Great Digestive Health.* New York, NY: Rodale, 2011. 124. Print.

Mullin, Gerard E., and Kathie Madonna. Swift. *The inside Tract: Your Good Gut Guide to Great Digestive Health.* New York, NY: Rodale, 2011. 40+. Print.

Murphree, R. "Yeast Overgrowth." *TreatingandBeating.com.* N.p., n.d. Web. 01 Apr. 2012. <http://drrodgermurphree.com/yeast-overgrowth/>.

Osborne, P. "The Gluten Sensitivity Spectrum." *SpectraCell Laboratories.* N.p., 2011. Web. 31 Mar. 2012. <http://www.spectracell.com/webinar-the-gluten-sensitivity-spectrum/>.

Pick, M. "Emotional Wellness: An Often Overlooked but Vital Component of Hormonal Balance." *Women to Women: The Personal Program for Hormonal Imbalance*. By D. Mills. Portland: Women to Women's Personal Program, 2008. 44-48. Print.

Schneider, Edward L., and Leigh Ann. Hirschman. "Making Menopause More Comfortable." *What Your Doctor Hasn't Told You and the Health-store Clerk Doesn't Know: The Truth about Alternative Treatments and What Works*. New York: Avery, 2006. 128-30. Print.

Seksik, P. "Gut Microbiota and IBD☆." *Gastroentérologie Clinique Et Biologique* 34.1 (2010): 44-51. Print.

Shames, Richard, and Karilee Halo. Shames. "Use Signs, Symptoms, and Family History to Support a Diagnosis." *Thyroid Power: Ten Steps to Total Health*. New York, NY: Harper Resource, 2001. 51-58. Print.

Simpson, Kathryn R. *Overcoming Adrenal Fatigue: How to Restore Hormonal Balance and Feel Renewed, Energized, and Stress Free*. Oakland, CA: New Harbinger Publications, 2011. Print.

Steinman, H. "Reproducibility of the ALCAT Test." *ALCAT Test*. N.p., n.d. Web. 31 Mar. 2012. <http://www.alcat.com/Images/Pdf/Reproducibility_of_the_ALCAT_Test.pdf>.

Talbott, S. "Dietary Supplements for Stress Adaptation." *The Cortisol Connection: Why Stress Makes You Fat and Ruins Your Health--and What You Can Do about It*. Second ed.

Alameda: Hunter House, 2007. 218-27. Print.

Teitelbaum, Jacob. "I-Infections: Destroy Your Body's Hidden Invaders." *From Fatigued to Fantastic!: A Clinically Proven Program to Regain Vibrant Health and Overcome Chronic Fatigue and Fibromyalgia.* New York: Avery, 2007. 133-34. Print.

Vojdani, A. "Why Test for Food IgA + IgM Antibody in Saliva IgA and IgG in Blood?" *BioHealth Diagnostics.* N.p., n.d. Web. 31 Mar. 2012. <http://intestinalbarriertst.com/pdf/Function-Intestinal-Barrier.pdf>.

Watson, B. "The Healthy Digestive System." *The H.O.P.E. Formula: The Ultimate Health Secret.* Clearwater: Renew Life and Information Services, 2006. 5-13. Print.

Weil, Andrew. "Disease Prevention: The Sustainable Solution." *Why Our Health Matters: A Vision of Medicine That Can Transform Our Future.* New York: Hudson Street, 2009. 138-43. Print.

Chapter 8: Change

Aschwanden, C. "Six Steps That Change Your Life." *Webmd.com.* N.p., n.d. Web. 29 Apr. 2012. <http://www.webmd.com/fitness-exercise/features/six-steps-that-can-change-your-life.>.

Chapter 9: Tree of Life

Cherry, K. "Hierarchy Of Needs." *About.com Psychology*. N.p., n.d. Web. 11 Aug. 2012. <http://psychology.about.com/od/theoriesofpersonality/a/hierarchyneeds.htm>.

Craig, Gary. "What Is EFT? - Theory, Science and Uses." *Garythink.com*. N.p., n.d. Web. 19 Aug. 2012. <http://www.garythink.com/eft/whatiseft.html>.

Dossey, Barbara Montgomery., Lynn Keegan, Cathie E. Guzzetta, and L. Gooding-Kolkmeier. *Holistic Nursing: A Handbook for Practice*. Second ed. Gaithersburg, MD: Aspen, 2000. Print.

Dossey, Barbara Montgomery., Lynn Keegan, Cathie E. Guzzetta, and Leslie Gooding-Kolkmeier. *Holistic Nursing: A Handbook for Practice*. Second ed. Gaithersburg, MD: Aspen, 1995. Print.

Hyman, M. "I Highly Recommend Meditation, and This Makes It Easy." 02 May 2012. E-mail.

Mehta, A. "Best Chakra Balancing Visualization Meditation Technique." *Mysticnaturals.com*. N.p., n.d. Web. 19 Aug. 2012. <http://secretgarden.mysticnaturals.com/articles/chakramed itation.htm>.

Morris, Joyce J., and William R. Morris. *Reiki: Hands That Heal*. York Beach, Me.: S. Weiser, 1999. Print.

Northrup, Christiane. "The Female Energy System." *Women's Bodies, Women's Wisdom: Creating Physical and Emotional Health and Healing.* Third ed. New York: Bantam, 2006. 74-97. Print.

Orloff, Judith. "Creating Positive Relationships and Combating Energy Vampires." *Positive Energy: 10 Extraordinary Prescriptions for Transforming Fatigue, Stress, and Fear into Vibrance, Strength, and Love.* New York: Harmony, 2004. 262-84. Print.

Phillips, B. *Where Science Meets Spirit: The Formula for Miracles.* N.p.: n.p., n.d. 2008. Web. 01 Aug. 2012.

Prout, Linda. "A Fresh Perspective: Balancing Who You Are with What You Eat." *Live in the Balance: The Ground-breaking East-West Nutrition Program.* New York: Marlowe &, 2000. 18-19. Print.

"Theta Healing." *Theta Healing Â Science.* N.p., n.d. Web. 01 Sept. 2012. <http://www.thetahealingtechnique.com/>.

"What Is Healing Touch?" *Healingtouchprogram.com.* N.p., n.d. Web. 01 Sept. 2012. <http://www.healingtouchprogram.com/about-healing-touch-program/what-is-healing-touch>.

"What Is Qi Gong?" *Exercisetoheal.com.* N.p., n.d. Web. 02 Sept. 2012. <http://www.exercisetoheal.com/What+Is+Qi+Gong%3F.html>.

"What Is Quantum Touch?" *Quantumtouch.com*. N.p., n.d. Web. 02 Sept. 2012.

<http://www.quantumtouch.com/index.php?option=com_content&view=article&id=3&It emid=58>.

Chapter 10: Transformation

Choquette, S. *Vitamins for the Soul: Daily Doses of Wisdom for Personal Empowerment*. Carlsbad, CA: Hay House, 2005. Print.

Index

5-HTP, 31
2-Hydroxyestrone, 169
16-Hydroxyestrone, 169
5-Hydroxy-L-Tryptophan, 31

A

Acidophilus, 105-106
Acid rain, 38-39
Action, 181, 186
Acupuncture, 134
Adaptogens, 174
Adenosine triphosphate, 99
Adrenal, 157
Adrenal fatigue, 151, 162
Adrenal glands, 23, 26, 159-160, 162, 175
Adrenal support, 174
Aerobic activity, 56-57
Air pollution, 36, 44-45
Aldosterone, 160, 162
Alpha brain waves, 21
Alpha lipoic acid, 98

American Pharmacists Association, 91
Amino acids, 75
Amylopectin A, 72
Androgen hormones, 159
Andropause, 166
Antibiotic, 103, 106, 110, 116
Anxiety, 31-32, 54
Arnica gel, 113
Ascorbic acid, 96
Ashwaganda, 174
ATP, 99
Aware, 14

B

Beneficial bacteria, 103, 138
Bifidobacteria, 103, 105-106
Biotin, 95
Bisphenol A, 40
Blood sugar, 21, 24, 65, 67, 70-71, 98
BMI, 53
Body mass index, 534

Botanical, 106-107
BPA, 40-41
Brain-derived
    Neurotrophic factor
    55

C

Calcium, 96, 99-100
Calcium citrate, 100
Calcium D-glucarate, 169
Candida, 141, 145-146
Celiac disease, 143
Center for Food Safety and
    Applied Nutrition, 89
Chakra, 14, 196-201, 203-
    204
Change, 179-180, 182, 187-
    188
Chaste berry, 169
Chia seeds, 101
Chinese ginseng, 174
Chlorella, 108
Chlorination, 41
Cholesterol, 40, 55, 67, 74,
    80, 94-95, 104, 158, 160,
Chromium, 38, 98

Chyme, 137
Circadian rhythm, 23, 26, 30,
    161
Clean Air Act, 44
Coconut oil, 82-83
Consumer Lab, 91, 108
Contemplation, 181, 184-185
Copper, 98-99
Cordyceps sinensis, 173
Cortisol, 23, 26, 122, 159-
    161, 163-164
C potency, 113, 171
Crown chakra, 199, 203

D

Delta brain waves, 21, 23
Dehyydroepiandroesterone,
    159
Detoxification, 136, 151-152,
    154-155
Detoxification program, 153
DHA, 102
DHEA, 159-160, 163-164,
    166, 173
Diabetes, 24, 62, 66-67
Diet, 62-63, 67, 159

Dietary Supplement and
  Nonprescription Drug
  Consumer Protection Act,
  90
Dietary Supplement Health
  and Education Act, 87, 89
Dietary Supplement
  Information Bureau, 87
Dietary Supplement
  Verification Program, 90-
  91
Digestive enzymes, 136, 147
Digestive tract, 136
Diindolymethane, 169
DIM, 169
Disease, 11, 16017
Docosahexaenoic acid, 102
Dopamine, 56
DSHEA, 87, 89
Dysbiosis, 139

E
EFA, 101-102
EFT, 134, 201, 205-206
Eicosapentaenoic acid, 102
Electromagnetic field, 37, 48, 155
Eleuthercoccus senticosus, 174
EMF, 48-50
Emotional blocks, 15, 127-130, 159, 207-208, 217
Emotional Freedom
  Technique, 134, 204-205
Emotions, 124-125, 131, 133, 161, 185, 205
Endocrine system, 46, 157
Endorphins, 55
Energy healing, 201, 211
Environment, 36
Environmental health, 36, 38
Environmental Protection
  Agency, 37
EPA, 37
Epinephrine, 162
Essential fatty acids, 101
Essential oils, 33, 107, 109-110
Estradiol, 164-165, 169, 172
Estriol, 164-165
Estrogen, 54, 159-160, 164-165

Estrogen disruptors, 47
Estrogen dominance, 160-161, 165-166, 168
Estrone, 164-165, 172
Eurycoma longiflora, 173
Exercise, 52, 54, 56-57, 155
Exercise benefits, 52, 54-55

F

Fast metabolizer, 152
Fat-soluable vitamins, 94, 96
Fatty liver, 67, 104
FDA, 73, 89
Fear, 12, 180, 217
Fish oil, 101-102
Five element theory, 125-126, 130, 161
Flax seed, 101
Fluoridation, 42-43
Fluoride, 41-43
Fluorosis, 42
Folate, 95
Food and Drug Administration, 73, 89
Food sensitivity, 70-72, 141-142, 146, 148, 151

Four laws, 194
Functional medicine, 17-18, 213-214
Functional testing, 30, 50

G

GABA, 31, 54
GALT, 138, 149
Gamma-amino butyric acid, 31
Gastrointestinal, 14, 18, 72, 104, 118, 123, 138, 140, 150-151, 176
Gastrointestinal flora, 138
Genetically modified, 36, 72-73, 84
Ginseng, 174
Glucocorticoids, 159, 161
Glucoronidase, 169
Glucose, 24
Glutathione pathway, 175
Glutathione peroxidase, 99
Gluten, 72, 143-145
Gluten sensitivity, 72, 143-144
GMO, 72-74, 84

GMP, 91
Good Manufacturing
   Practice, 91
Gratitude, 13, 15, 132-133
Gut-associated lymphoid
   Tissue, 138, 149
Glycemic index, 67-68

H
Hatha yoga, 58
Healing, 14-16
Healing touch, 121-122, 134,
   201, 208, 210
Health, 122, 213
Health care, 120, 213
Heart chakra, 198-199, 203-
   204
Heavy metal toxicity, 39-40
Hemp seeds, 101
HEPA, 46
Herbal, 93, 106-107
Herxheimer reaction, 147
High-efficiency Particulate
   Air, 46

Homeopathic medicines, 107,
   111-112, 170
Homeopathy, 93, 111-113,
   170-171, 173
H.O.P.E., 188
Hops, 32
Hormone, 156-157
Hormone Replacement
   Therapy, 167
HPA axis, 122, 158, 162, 174
HRT, 167
Human growth hormone, 54,
   159
Hyperthyroidism, 163
Hypothalamus-pituitary-
   Adrenal axis, 122, 158
Hypothyroidism, 42, 139,
   144, 163, 165

I
Ig A, 142
Ig E, 142
Ig G, 142
Illness, 7, 11, 18
Indian ginseng, 174
Indole-3-carbinole, 168-169
Inflammation, 24, 41, 67, 70,

72, 75, 108, 143, 150, 159
Insulin, 23-24, 159, 162
Insulin resistance, 24, 67, 162
Intestinal permeability, 112, 138, 148
Iodine, 98-99, 175

K
Karma, 193
Krill oil, 102

L
Lactobacillus, 103, 105-106
Large intestine, 137
Lauric acid, 82
Lavender, 33
Leaky gut syndrome, 148
Leukocyte reactivity, 142
LM potency, 113, 172
Long chain fatty acids, 82
L-Tyrosine, 175
Lyon Diet Heart Study, 66

M
Magnesium, 181, 187
Maintenance, 181, 187
Maslow's Hierarchy of Needs, 190, 192
Massage, 16, 134
Meditation, 121, 134, 202-204
Mediterranean diet, 64-65, 67-68, 70, 81
Medium chain fatty acids, 82
Melatonin, 26-27, 30-31, 49
Menopause, 144, 160, 165, 173
Mercury toxicity, 101
Microalgae oil, 102
Mineralcorticoids, 159
Minerals, 74-75, 87, 93, 98
Monolaurin, 83
Monounsaturated fats, 80-81
M potency, 113, 172
Mucosal barrier, 138-140, 148

N

Narcolepsy, 29
National Center of Complementary and Alternative Medicine, 90
National Institutes of Health, 90, 210
Natural Products Association Good Manufacturing Practices Certification Program, 91
Natural Standards Database, 108
NCCAM, 90
Niacin, 94
NIH, 90
Nirvana, 218
Non-rapid eye movement, 21
Norepinephrine, 55, 122, 162
NREM, 21, 22
NSF International Dietary Supplements Certification Program, 91
Nursing, 5

O

Office of Cancer Complementary and Alternative Medicine, 90
Office of Dietary Supplements, 90
Omega-3-fatty acids, 81, 102-103
Organic, 84
Oscillococcinum, 112-113
Oxidation, 41

P

Panax ginseng, 174
Pantothenic acid, 95
Parabens, 47
Parasites, 141, 148-149
Parkinson's Disease, 39, 65
Passionflower, 32-33
Path to health, 6-7, 21, 181
Peripheral neuropathy, 28
Persistent organic pollutants, 46
Pesticides, 36, 38-39
Phosphatidyl-choline, 102
Phosphorus, 100

Pilates, 58
Pineal gland, 49
Pituitary, 157, 169
Polyunsaturated fats, 80-81
POP, 46
Potassium, 98-99
Potency, 112-113, 171
PNI, 122-123
Prayer, 193, 201-202
Pre-contemplation, 181-182
Pregnenolone, 160, 163
Preparation, 181, 185
Probiotic, 103-105, 139, 146
Prochaska's Theoretical Model for Change, 181-182
Progestagen, 159
Progesterone, 54, 159-161, 165, 168-169
Psychoneuroimmunology, 122, 208
Purpose, 12-13
Pyridoxine, 95

Q

Qi, 192-193, 196
Qi Gong, 134, 201, 211-212
Quantum physics, 206, 208
Quantum touch, 134, 201, 208-209

R

Radon, 45
Rapid eye movement, 21
Reiki, 134, 201, 208-209
Relaxation, 122-123, 209
Relaxation techniques, 134
REM, 21-22
Restless leg syndrome, 28-29, 139
Rhodiola rosea, 174
Riboflavin, 94
Root chakra, 197, 203-204
Root of illness, 7

S

Saccharomyces boulardii, 105-106
Sacral chakra, 197, 203-204
S.A.D. , 36

Saliva testing, 50, 168
Saturated fats, 80-81
Secretory IgA, 139-141, 149-151, 164
Seed 4 Change, 7, 20
Selenium, 46, 98-99, 175
Self-transformation, 192-193, 217
Serotonin, 31, 55, 104
Siberian ginseng, 174
Simillimum, 112, 171
Sleep, 20-21, 117
Sleep apnea, 28
Sleep deprivation, 22, 24
Sleep disorder, 28-29
Sleep habits, 25-26
Sleep hygiene, 26-27
Slow metabolizer, 152
Small intestine, 137
Sodium, 98-99
Solar plexus chakra, 198, 203-204
Spiritual, 119-120, 193
Spirituality, 119-120, 122
Standard American Diet, 36
Steroidal hormone

Principal pathways, 158
Stress, 24, 55, 67, 118-119, 123, 131, 133, 159, 161, 211
Succussion, 112, 170
Supplements, 87-89, 92-93, 114

T

Tai chi, 134, 201, 211-212
T-cell, 24
Termination, 181, 187
Testosterone, 54, 160, 164, 166, 173
The China Study, 68-69
Theta brainwaves, 207-208
Theta healing, 201, 206-208
Thiamine, 94
Third eye chakra, 199, 203-204
Throat chakra, 199, 203-204
Thyroid gland, 163
Thyroid hormone, 157, 159, 162-163, 175

Traditional Chinese Medicine, 125, 152, 192
Trans-fatty, 80
Transformation, 14, 133, 182
Tree of Life, 7, 14, 19, 190-192, 216-218
Turmeric, 108

U
USP, 90
U.S. Pharmacopia, 90

V
Valerian, 32
Villi, 137, 139-140
Vitamin, 74-75, 87, 93, 104
Vitamin A, 94, 96, 100
Vitamin B1, 94
Vitamin B2, 94
Vitamin B3, 94
Vitamin B5, 95
Vitamin B6, 95
Vitamin B7, 95
Vitamin B9, 95
Vitamin B12, 95
Vitamin C, 46, 94, 96
Vitamin D, 94, 96-97
Vitamin E, 94, 96
Vitamin K, 94, 96-97, 100, 104
VOC, 45
Volatile organic compounds, 45

W
Walnuts, 102
Water-soluable vitamins, 94
WHI, 167
Women's Health Initiative Study, 167

X
Xenobiotics, 46
X potency, 113, 171

Y
Yeast overgrowth, 145-146
Yoga, 134, 201, 211-212

Z
Zinc, 98-99

www.pathtohealthandhealing.com

Made in the USA
Lexington, KY
22 August 2015